EN

This book is a must for older folks involved in or contemplating a new relationship. It is eminently readable, filled with wise comments and suggestions interspersed with lively stories of couples who have found love in later life.

Marjorie Wood, Ph.D.
Founding President of the East Bay (California) chapter of the Association of Marriage and Family Counselors.

Older Couples: New Couplings is a welcome resource for older adults who are in, or thinking about, forming new relationships. Based on extensive interviews, it offers interesting and helpful insights into the complex process of finding and nurturing new partnerships. Demonstrating that it's never too late, this book provides a unique look at the ageless wonder of becoming a couple again.

Barrie Robinson, MSW
Gerontology Lecturer, School of Social Welfare,
University of California, Berkeley

A fascinating book, depicting the many different types of newly-formed love relationships experienced by elders. This is an excellent resource, not only for older folks and their concerned children but for classes studying the sociology of aging.

Dr. Glen Caspers Doyle, Professor
Interdisciplinary Gerontology Program, College of Health and Human Service, California State University, Fresno

COMMENTS FROM OUR READERS

We're happily married and can identify with many of the couples described in this book. It reaffirms and reinforces the enjoyable way we conduct our life together. Every older couple should read it ... they can learn from it.

AE, Walnut Creek, California

My husband and I, in our sixties, have been together for six months. We have many arguments and differences. Your book has enabled us to better understand each other and work things out. The experiences of many couples, along with useful suggestions, make this a valuable reading.

DW, Oakhurst, California

My dad died two years ago and my mother has been lonely ever since. When I showed her your book she became interested in finding a new relationship. Tonight she has her third date! The section on *How Do You Find a Partner?* was particularly helpful to her.

RF, Sacramento, California

My mother passed away over a year ago and my father now is involved with another woman. I wanted no one to take my mother's place and I was jealous of the time my father spent with his new love. Reading your book has helped me to accept his new relationship, and the three of us get along much better now.

TL, San Jose, California

You say your book is for older couples. I am 41 and my new husband is 44. Boy, has your book been helpful to us! It should be read by any couple starting a second relationship.

SZ, Monterey, California

Older Couples:

New Couplings

Finding and Keeping Love in Later Life

Edith Ankersmit Kemp, L.C.S.W.

Jerrold E. Kemp, Ed.D.

Unlimited Publishing

Bloomington, Indiana

Distributing Publisher:
Unlimited Publishing, LLC
Bloomington, Indiana
http://www.unlimitedpublishing.com

Cover and Book Design by Charles King

ISBN 1-58832-019-7

Unlimited Publishing

Bloomington, Indiana

According to the *Lummis* [an Indian tribe], old age was the proper time to fall in love. Old age was the proper time to suffer romances, and jealousy, and lose your head—old age, when you felt things more, and could spare the time to go dead nuts over a person, and understand how fine a thing it was. This is how the *Lummis* saw it.

Annie Dillard, *The Living* (1992); New York, HarperCollins, page 101

CONTENTS

Section Two: IMPORTANT TOPICS FOR OLDER COUPLES

Section Three: HOW DO YOU FIND A PARTNER?

Section Four: USEFUL INFORMATION FOR OLDER INDIVIDUALS AND COUPLES

ACKNOWLEDGEMENTS

Thanks to Judith Wallerstein, whose book *The Good Marriage,* gave us the inspiration for this project. Acknowledgement to James Landers for his literature search that found no book dealing with relationships formed in later life. Our gratitude to Rachel Oliver, psychologist, who interviewed us so that we could experience the process before Edith interviewed others. We owe our greatest debt to the couples who so freely shared their joys and struggles. Their strong motivation was a desire to help others in similar situations. To ensure privacy, their names and other identifying information have been changed.

We wish to recognize those professional colleagues who reviewed our book, many of whom provided helpful suggestions. They include Midge Wood, Pat Spohn, Blanche Jaggi, Jaqueline Ensign, Vera Lis, Jane Loebel, Barbara Leff, Jay Thorwaldson, Barrie Robinson, Glen Doyle, and Judith Wallerstein.

Thanks to Kristina Rylands for her assistance in editing and in choosing themes for the interview chapters; estate attorney Lynn Rice, who consulted with us to ensure the accuracy of the chapter dealing with legal matters; Muriel Warren, for the photograph appearing on the cover of this book; and Denise Metzger, Accent on Words, who handled the final editing and formatting of the manuscript for the publisher.

Edith Ankersmit Kemp and Jerry Kemp

Preface

SETTING THE STAGE

We, Edith Ankersmit Kemp and Jerry Kemp, the authors of this book, were introduced to each other by mutual friends. Jerry was 75. His wife died a year and a half earlier, and Edith, age 66, had been a widow for four years. Both of our spouses had long illnesses prior to their deaths. No more than a month passed before we knew we loved each other, and living a three-hour drive apart, we visited as often as we could.

Nine months after we met, Edith moved from her urban home to Jerry's country home. She brought in some of her furniture and changed almost everything on the walls. The house was dark, so we installed skylights in the roof. Jerry knew she wanted as much as possible to make it *our* home, and he went along with her changes. The decorations he likes best are the ones we bought *together.*

In that first year of living together, we enjoyed sharing activities such as hiking, square dancing, watching Public Television programs together, and visiting each other's friends. Our life was full of fun, joy, passion (yes, at our ages!), and a lot of adjustments. Our different habits formed over many years of life without each other have caused the most conflicts. Edith forgot to turn off lights and close the toilet seat cover, both of which habits "bugged" Jerry to no end. Jerry is extremely punctual, and we had some blow ups about Edith keeping him waiting. When she first moved in, every table surface was covered with papers, journals, and books. Dust and cobwebs were everywhere. Edith has since learned to be more punctual, and now Jerry strives to keep the house clean and neat, except for his desk, which we've agreed can stay a mess. Edith still forgets a light sometimes, but Jerry just turns it off. Some things still bother him, but he keeps his mouth shut. (Edith hates being lectured and he knows it.)

A year after starting to live together, we married. Though we are still making adjustments, and will be doing so for the rest of our lives, our time together is much smoother. We began to wonder how other older couples forming new relationships made their adjustments. What habits did they change? How did they learn to accept, or at least tolerate, each other's behaviors? What about finances, health, sexuality, hobbies, eating habits, entertainment, and relationships with children and grandchildren?

These questions piqued our curiosity. Edith is a licensed psychotherapist, and has worked with couples for many years. She has helped them examine the patterns in their relationships and find ways to improve their interactions, often saving a troubled marriage. Jerry is the author of three textbooks in his field and has brought his writing and organizational skills to this book. Now, as partners in a newly formed older-couple relationship, we wanted to discover how other older couples think, deal with their problems, and make their decisions. Our plan was to offer persons who are either involved in an older-couple relationship or contemplating one, the opportunity to learn from others in similar situations. We also desired to provide practical advice and suggestions that our readers could apply to their own lives.

Our inspiration was Judith Wallerstein's thoughtful book, *The Good Marriage*. Of the many couples she interviewed, the only older pair had been together since their early twenties. We searched and found little written about older couples forming new relationships.

We know that people are now living longer, leading to the potential for more older individuals to form new relationships. This conclusion is supported by these statistics:

- From 1980 to 2000, the number of persons 65 years of age and older in the United States will have increased by nine million.

- From 1980 to 1996, the number of widowed and divorced seniors increased by 14.3% (*Statistical Abstract of the United States* (1997); Bureau of the Census. Washington, DC, Table 47, page 48)

Today's senior citizens are healthier, more active, and receive better medical attention than ever before. Therefore, it can be expected that older people will be more likely to want to form new relationships, enjoying their remaining years in pleasurable sharing.

As we prepared to locate potential couples to interview, we recognized the different arrangements that people make today in their associations. Therefore, we sought couples either married, living together, or living separately but in a committed relationship. We required at least one partner to be over age 55 when their relationship started and that they had been together for at least a year so there would be time to experience problems and make adjustments. We have included a number of couples who had been together for many years. This allowed us to examine the changes taking place over time with increasing age.

To attract couples for the book, we publicized in urban, suburban, and rural areas in Northern California. An article about our project was published in local newspapers and in newsletters of retirement communities. As a result, we received offers from many couples who wanted to participate, and we contacted those who fit our criteria. Based on Edith's more than 25 years of experience as a counselor, she conducted the interviews.

This is an anecdotal rather than a statistical study. We do not claim to measure the success or failure of late-life marriages in any particular population. Our sample is small and self-selected. Most of our couples were "tickled pink" with their relationship and wanted to share their stories. (Naturally, they all experienced some problems and had adjustments to make.) We attempted to interest minority couples in being interviewed; unfortunately with no success. We do however, cover a wide range of locations, ages, backgrounds, and approaches to life. We believe that you will find the stories of those interviewed to be encouraging, and that their experiences and Edith's suggestions will be useful in your life.

During the interviews, Edith asked a range of questions including: *How did you meet? What attracted you to each other? How did your relationship develop? What kinds of problems did you face and what adjustments did you make?* Each person provided information about his or her family history, previous relationships, religious practices, financial arrangements, and health and sexuality. Edith also wanted to get a glimpse into what their daily lives were like.

Generally, there were three interview sessions. Usually Edith visited with each partner separately in the couple's home or in their separate homes. She then interviewed the two jointly. Occasionally, when appropriate, she only met with a couple together. A complete interview lasted from three to five hours and was recorded on tape. Suitably long visits were important in order to get a feel for each individual in his or her surroundings and the quality of the couple's relationship. We very much appreciate the openness of those who cooperated and believe the experience was enjoyable and often beneficial to the participants.

Some of the topics discussed with each person revealed differences that were reviewed in the third session together. This joint interview helped Edith gain a sense of the nature of the interaction between the pair. At times, the couple used this session to understand their own differences better. On the other hand, this experience often made the two persons more aware of particularly good relations they had established between themselves. One couple said, "This interview is reminding us of how much we love each other."

Section One of the book, *Introducing Our Couples,* consists of summaries of interviews with 15 couples, using fictitious names and changing identifying information to protect their privacy.

Once you are introduced to the couples, continue to Section Two, which treats *Important Topics for Older Couples.* Here you will find and recognize each couple again as their experiences are described in six topic chapters.

If you might be interested in starting a new relationship yourself but not know how to go about the process, Section Three provides useful answers to the question, *How Do You Find a Partner?* It consists of three chapters, with examples from the couples interviewed.

Section Four summarizes *Useful Information for Older Individuals and Couples,* relating to two major subjects that you might not know how to manage best.

We came to this study with a mindset that older couples might have serious difficulties in adjusting because of the partners' many years of forming different habits, either alone or with a previous mate. To our surprise, we found a great deal more positive than negative responses. Many couples reported that they now have more joy, more freedom, enhanced affection, and better sexuality than they found in their earlier relationships. This was true for those who were widowed as well as for those who had been divorced.

Why is this so? We discovered a number of possible reasons for these enriched late-in-life relationships. For example, with long-life experiences, many of them painful, comes a greater maturity and appreciation for the essentials in life, as does the awareness that with age, time is limited. Also, there are no longer children to raise, and with most individuals, no jobs to go to with demanding work schedules and difficult responsibilities. This allows more time and energy for new partners to enjoy each other. To avoid the irritability that can result from too much time together, we found that most couples interviewed arranged for some degree of separateness. This ranges from living apart to finding private places in the same house, and engaging in individual activities at times.

Following are a few principles that the couples interviewed have taught us. The chapters describing each couple, and the topical subject chapters, will bring these principles to life.

- Later in life an individual's beliefs, lifestyle, and habits are more set. Some adjustments can be made, but the primary key to a good relationship is acceptance of your partner as he or she is.

- Sexual satisfaction is possible throughout life. Age is no barrier.

- Adult children may or may not be pleased with the new relationship. If unfortunately, they are not, it is important to keep your commitment to each other primary.

- Financial arrangements need to be discussed early in your relationship, with particular attention given to how expenses will be shared.

- Be aware that as your partner ages, you may become a caretaker. It is normal to have some feelings of resentment. As long as your actions express care and affection, you need not blame yourself for your feelings.

The final chapter of this book—*Concluding Thoughts*—restates the above principles and others derived from the content. Also, here are Edith's general observations and insights. Some of these deal with human development and how it relates to the formation of intimate relationships, particularly those of older couples. We hope this will give a wider perspective to the content in the preceding chapters.

The book ends with two indexes. The *Interviewee Index* lists pages on which references are made to each person interviewed. The *Topical Index* contains references to the many subjects treated in chapters of Sections Two, Three and Four.

Whether you are an older person contemplating the start of a relationship or you are in a relationship that is having difficulties, this book can provide some insight and suggestions. It can also reinforce the successful practices of those couples who are well adjusted and happy. Support persons, including adult children, senior-center counselors, bereavement professionals, and geriatric instructors can all benefit from this book.

Every effort has been made to keep confidential the identities of the couples interviewed without losing the full flavor and nature of their relationship. We owe a great deal to those who so freely shared their intimate thoughts, feelings, and experiences with Edith, in the hopes that they could be helpful to other older folks embarking on a new love and a new life together.

Edith Ankersmit Kemp and Jerrold E. Kemp

Section One

INTRODUCING OUR COUPLES

This Section consists of information gathered during Edith's interviews with 15 couples. Fictitious names are used, and identifying information is changed to protect the privacy of the couples. Each chapter begins with the statement of a theme that speaks to an issue that this particular couple exemplifies. Then, by reading their answers to the questions Edith asked, you intimately meet each couple. With some topics, we refer to couples discussed in other chapters of this Section. Each time, their names appear in **boldface**.

Interspersed in the interviews are indented statements proceeded by an asterisk (*). These are Edith's observations, which point out important principles or practices. They are based on both her knowledge as a psychotherapist and her personal experience as a widow who has formed a fulfilling new relationship. We hope that a look into the lives of these couples, seeing both their joys and struggles, along with Edith's analyses and comments, will be beneficial to you.

If you are interested in following further experiences of any of the 15 couples described in these chapters, see their **boldfaced** names in the content of chapters in Sections Two and Three. The names are also listed in the Interviewee Index, with references to each entry in the book.

Chapter 1

(Interview: Joanne and Andy)

LIFE IS SHORT ... EAT DESSERT FIRST

He's an intellectual. She's a woman with a showgirl personality. She likes rock music; he's into classical. They're attractive, intelligent, and deeply in love. Both have been divorced and have gone through hard times. In their new relationship, they are learning to compromise and to share while each still maintains a distinct individuality.

THEME
Balancing Separateness and Togetherness

Joanne and Andy illustrate a universal theme in all relationships—maintaining a balance between separateness and togetherness. This is especially important with couples who have had many years of living separate lives with different habits and interests. They are most articulate about this theme. They also demonstrate how individuals can grow throughout life and how pain from the past can lead to treasuring the moment and their present relationship.

INTRODUCING JOANNE AND ANDY

Joanne is 59 and Andy is 60. They rent an apartment in the center of a busy city with high-rise buildings, shopping centers, and congested traffic. They had begun dating 14 months earlier and have been living together for 8 months. When I arrived, Andy was out on an errand. Joanne graciously ushered me into their spacious and elegantly furnished apartment.

Joanne looks much younger than her years. She has stylishly cut black hair and is very attractive, outgoing, and articulate. Andy, who arrived later, is a husky, balding man with warm, brown eyes. He was slower to warm up in conversation than was Joanne, but he gradually relaxed, became candid and outgoing; he had a sparkle in his eyes, and an engaging smile.

HOW DID YOU MEET?

Joanne was vice president in charge of marketing for a large corporation. One afternoon she was walking through her building and approached a company accountant she had casually known only on a "hello" basis. He was standing with someone talking about jazz. As Joanne passed, she flippantly said "93.6" (the FM frequency for the local jazz radio station). This remark caught Andy's attention. Thereafter, when they saw each other, they would say little things about jazz to each other.

Then one day when Joanne saw Andy in the lunchroom, she sneezed, and he said, "Bless you, my child." "Thank you Father," Joanne replied. He asked, "Are you of that ilk?" "I was," she responded. Andy invited Joanne to his office "to talk about it." They discovered each had been raised Catholic, and after a little chat, he asked her to attend a jazz concert with him. Thus began their dating.

HOW WERE YOU ATTRACTED TO EACH OTHER?

When Andy first noticed Joanne, he was caught by her walk, which showed a jaunty spirit and a lively bounce. Immediately interested, he looked her up in the company's employee database, finding her age and marital status.

What had attracted Joanne? "Trust was a big issue with me, and I trusted Andy almost from the beginning. He's the first man I've wanted to hold hands with while walking down the street. I feel trusting and at peace with him."

> * Joanne had enough life experience to sense that trust can be one of the most important features of any relationship. Young people often are drawn together by physical features. Many older persons, having experienced difficulties, as Joanne had in the past, recognize that basic integrity is more important.
>
> In my counseling with couples, I also see integrity as a key factor. If the basic love, care, and sense of responsibility exists, I have hope that, with help, differences can be resolved. Joanne, sensing Andy's trustworthiness, has been willing to work out many small disagreements between them.

HOW DID YOUR RELATIONSHIP DEVELOP?

Joanne and Andy began living together when she left the company to start her own consulting business and he retired. They both moved from their separate apartments to a larger one where they each could have separate spaces. They also have individual phone numbers and their own post office boxes. Most of the furniture was Joanne's. She told me that Andy "didn't have a home—he had a place to live. It looked like a motel room." Now the furniture is tasteful, and the apartment is meticulously neat, except for Andy's messy, separate room.

* Here we see very concrete examples of separateness—the spaces in the apartment, phone numbers, and post office boxes. The overall neatness of the apartment shows that, except for his own separate space, Andy adjusted and learned to keep the rest of the apartment tidy. In doing so, he recognized Joanne's need for neatness, and this compromise contributes to their togetherness.

WHAT WERE YOUR EARLY LIVES LIKE?

Joanne and Andy have similar childhood backgrounds. They both came from working-class Catholic families. Joanne's parents fought frequently, and her father was a volatile, alcoholic gambler. She was the eldest child and the "family peacemaker."

Andy was the second of seven children in a poor immigrant family. His father was a stern disciplinarian who frequently beat the four boys. Joanne and Andy believe that their similar upbringings helped bind them together.

WHAT WERE YOUR PREVIOUS RELATIONSHIPS LIKE?

Andy

Andy had a previous marriage that lasted 21 years of sullen non-communication and 10 years with no sex. He was never unfaithful and waited until their daughter was 18 before he left his wife.

* This is surely an example of Andy's basic integrity and trustworthiness. My husband Jerry, had a companionable marriage, but his wife, because of emotional difficulties and her long illness, had little interest in sex. He faithfully remained with her for 45 years until her death. This

> was an indication to me of Jerry's basic trustworthiness and integrity.

After their divorce, Andy had nine years of single life, during which time he was very active sexually. (Says Joanne on the side, "Like a rabbit!")

Joanne

Joanne was married for 23 years to her first husband and had two daughters. She had known her husband since she was 18 and describes the marriage as "loveless … not much affection, not good sex." She was a homemaker for many years but went back to school at age 35 for her college degree. Ultimately, it was she who left the marriage.

She was with her second husband for nine difficult years. He was a manic-depressive, had a violent temper, was verbally abusive, threw things, and on several occasions, struck her in anger. One day, after taking a shower, she went into the garage and found him dead, hanging from the vacuum cleaner cord. This tragedy, along with other losses, including deaths in the family and children moving away, left her with "a hole in my heart as big as a Mack truck" and skittish about forming a new relationship.

She was then involved for four years with a wealthy man who was 20 years her senior. She described that relationship as mainly a mutually supportive friendship (he had recently lost his wife) with occasional sex. She was still seeing him when she met Andy, and their parting was friendly.

> * Earlier we learned that Joanne was the eldest child and the family "peacemaker." A child in such a position, when becoming an adult, often assumes a caretaker role in

relationships. Joanne certainly did this with her second husband, but as much as she tried, she could not help him. Of course she then was cautious about forming a new relationship. Her union with this older man was not a deep involvement and was very much a safe haven after the intensity of her second marriage. Because she was not deeply in love, she felt safe and was able to recover from the pain of her husband's suicide. It gave her time to be ready to love Andy.

HOW DO YOU BALANCE INTERESTS, HABITS, AND ACTIVITIES?

Joanne and Andy see themselves as "two circles coming together but still trying to keep our own identities." The way they balance their activities, allowing for both separate and quality together times, concretely shows how the two circles do come together, yet allowing them to keep their unique individualities.

Joanne likes almost any movie, while Andy prefers intellectual and foreign films. Sometimes they see a movie together, sometimes separately. Joanne enjoys a type of rock music that Andy doesn't care for, while he prefers to listen to classical selections. Other than good jazz, which they both like, they tolerate each other's music. They have three television sets in the apartment for *his – hers – our* programs. They eat together whenever possible and both were vegetarians before they met. Also, they take short walks, bicycle, and go to jazz concerts together.

Both Joanne and Andy have had to change several of their own habits while accepting some of their partner's. Andy was used to dropping his things on the floor, picking them up only if visitors came, and leaving the dishes in the sink until it was full. The first adjustment he made when they began to live together was with neatness. "I just did it," said Andy with pride. The day I visited, Joanne was about to leave for a two-week visit with her daughter. Andy knew the apartment would become a mess while she was gone, but he would rush to straighten it up before she returned. He lets himself go when he is alone, but he knows that Joanne wants a neat home and makes a real effort to please her.

Joanne also has habits that bother Andy. She often forgets to close the refrigerator. She sets her purse on the kitchen counter, although Andy is concerned it might have been on a dirty floor. Wisely, he doesn't make an issue of it.

Andy has a room of his own in their apartment where he keeps his clothes and other personal items. They sleep together in the master bedroom, but the closets in that room are for Joanne's use. They have separate bathrooms and Joanne laughed, "I think sharing a bathroom would have done in our relationship."

> * I like Joanne's humor. It is a saving factor in a relationship, especially with an older couple who have acquired so many different habits. I appreciate the way Joanne looks at the lighter side of sharing space with a partner. I like to joke with my couples in counseling. It helps them laugh at themselves. Jerry and I keep a spark lit between us with humor, thus greatly diffusing any conflict.

The issue of keeping his own identity is especially important to Andy. He explains, "One change that is happening to me in our relationship is that many of the things that were important to me in the past I have given up. I wonder if it's going to bite me someday. I don't know. The whole cycle of a relationship starts out with two people knocking themselves out to please one another. Then they gradually attempt to find what they want and take tentative steps to get it. That's about where I am now."

* Here Andy is particularly articulate about what older couples face because they have habits and ideas formed over many years. They must gradually find a balance between accommodating each other and holding on to what is especially important to each individual.

In tolerating each other's music when together, Joanne and Andy accommodate each other. By having their own television sets, they respect their different preferences and hold on to their own autonomy. In a happy relationship, partners both give up a little to please each other and maintain the basic tastes and values that are essential parts of themselves.

Jerry and I also have worked to balance autonomy and togetherness. Like Joanne and Andy, we have different tastes in music. Jerry likes big band and show music. I prefer classical. Neither of us objects to the other's music, so we listen to both kinds together. When I'm alone, I play ethnic music loud and sing along. Jerry listens to Cole Porter, George Gershwin, and Frank Sinatra when I'm gone. We enjoy hiking together, but I ski alone or with friends. I read novels, while he reads the daily newspaper and weekly news magazines. We both enjoy watching news commentary television and then discussing issues.

It is important to consider the following issues when balancing autonomy and togetherness: What can you do together? What can you, without resentment, allow your partner to enjoy separately? What habits can you change? What can you accept in your partner? Resolving these small issues is a good part of what makes a successful relationship.

WHAT MAKES THIS RELATIONSHIP WORK SO WELL?

When I saw Joanne and Andy together, the sparkle, humor, and affection between them was obvious. At one point Andy, looking at Joanne, said "You're everything I ever wanted. I'm not settling for less at all." Joanne laughed and blushed, saying, "How can I resist him?"

Then Andy, with sincerity said, "In Joanne I seem to have found most of the things I value in a person. She's attractive, sexual, bright, and competent. She doesn't take any crap from me, which I admire a lot. I can be a bully like my father. This woman can't be frightened. Our relationship is much more important than any disagreements we might have."

"I realize that we don't have forever in terms of time," Joanne continued. "We're not going to raise children together. I've been through menopause. We've come to a different place in our lives. It's nice to find a companion. See that little plaque up on the wall? '*Life's Uncertain, Eat Dessert First.*' I think we both have had life experiences that have made us realize what's really important, and we are willing to work on our relationship. Andy is a cancer survivor and went through a very tragic period in his life. My second husband committed suicide, and at that same period of time, everyone who was important to me left. When you experience so much sadness, I think you look at life differently. You want joy in living because life's very uncertain. So when you go through such traumas and survive, you're never quite the same. What might have been important then isn't important now. What I might have said before, I now hold back. If I could go back and relive my first marriage with the knowledge and experience I now have, I think even that might have succeeded."

* Like Joanne, with the loss of my husband and then of dear friends, I have gained a deeper appreciation of living in the present ... a thankfulness for each moment of each day. Now Jerry and I are keenly aware that our time is limited. We both have had, as did Joanne and Andy, much sadness in our lives. Therefore, every day of our new life together is a gift to savor. We do "eat dessert first."

As they are still in the relatively early stage of their relationship, they have concerns about long-term commitment. Joanne and Andy have slightly different perspectives. Joanne speaks frankly: "Andy talks about being together forever. I've had too many losses and unpleasant situations. I just want to live for now." She is afraid of the possessiveness and control that she sees as part of a marriage. If married, she fears she couldn't spend what she wanted, especially on clothes. She has asked Andy if he would be upset if she bought $2,000 worth of clothes, and he said that frankly, he would be annoyed.

Andy underscores his long-term commitment: "Recently, when we were on the airplane on our way to visit my mother, I knew Joanne was the most important person in my life and would remain so." On the other hand, Joanne believes, "We could be talking of living together for two years or for 20 years." They both talk about a long-term relationship, but are a little gun-shy. They use phrases such as: "We're going to make it through the day." "It's a-day-to-day thing." "We're still in the stage where we're hoping."

* Remember the short period of time they have been together (dating for 14 months and then living together for eight months). Also recall their very difficult previous relationships. It is understandable that they are still in the "hoping stage."

I said goodbye to Joanne and Andy as Joanne dashed off to a hair appointment, getting ready for a two-week trip to visit her daughter.

FINAL OBSERVATIONS

This couple is an excellent example of how to balance separateness and togetherness. In successfully doing this in the early stages of their relationship, I believe they are on their way to a long and happy union.

They also are an example of how difficult childhoods can at first lead to repeating painful early experiences in a marriage. Certainly Joanne did, choosing as her second husband a volatile, unstable, but perhaps exciting man, much like her father. I would presume that Andy walled himself off from being expressive and seeking affection because of his upbringing in a large family with a stern, physically abusive father. This led to his enduring a lengthy cold and distant marriage. But Joanne and Andy also are a shining example of how, in later years, by learning from the past, old patterns can be overcome. It is never too late to experience the sharing, love, and affection for which humans deeply long.

Chapter 2

(Interview: Ruth and Paul)

A SECOND LIFE WITH A NEW LOVE

After her first husband died, Ruth made up her mind not to get married again. Then a friend from long ago, whose first wife was entirely incapacitated with Alzheimer's disease, invited her to attend a conference with him. He mailed her an airline ticket, and enclosed a brochure from the hotel showing a picture of a guest room with a king-size bed. "What a presumptuous rascal," she thought. And so started a meaningful relationship leading to a happy marriage.

THEME
Renewing Life's Joy after Years of Caretaking

Caring for a seriously ill loved one over many years is so all-consuming that one can lose part of oneself. What a delight it must be to find yourself again with a new love. Life does go on and for Ruth and Paul, it did.

INTRODUCING RUTH AND PAUL

It was a trying 20 miles on a dusty dirt road to their home, and the drive seemed to take forever. The few house numbers on the road were confusing, and I thought I might be lost. I pulled up to a dilapidated old trailer and was told that Ruth and Paul lived just down the road. Sure enough, there was their house number a short drive farther. I climbed a hill to find, to my surprise after all that heat and dust, a large redwood house surrounded by a lovely garden. Both Ruth and Paul came to the door to greet me. Ruth is a tall slender woman with short gray hair and blue eyes sparkling in her pleasantly wrinkled face. Paul is a handsome man of medium build, slightly heavy, with a warm smile. They were both dressed in carefully pressed pants and shirts. We made ourselves comfortable around the kitchen table, and our interview began.

Ruth is 78 years old and Paul is 80. They have been married seven years, and both had been widowed. They live on a ranch that originally belonged to Ruth and her first husband. After our interview, Ruth and Paul gave me a tour of the house and grounds. Their house is spacious and comfortable. When they decided that Paul would join Ruth in her home, they had the bedroom enlarged with a new bathroom, and a large closet added for Paul's clothes.

On the grounds are large flower and vegetable gardens and a barn with a corral for animals. The house furnishings are of oriental design, and I was interested to see a striking silk tapestry of a Japanese ceremony.

HOW DID YOU MEET?

During World War II, Paul, Ruth, and her first husband all worked for the same defense company. Ruth was in a clerical position, her husband was a machinist, and Paul, among other responsibilities, was in quality control. The two couples (Ruth and her husband, and Paul and his wife) met at a social gathering, and their friendship began. They often had dinner together, enjoying each other's company.

Then Paul entered military service, while Ruth and her husband continued their employment in the defense company for a total of 15 years. The two couples kept in contact, particularly through the exchange of Christmas cards and letters, though because of distance, they no longer visited each other. In 1970, Paul, who owned a building-supply company, provided Ruth and her husband with supplies to renovate their newly purchased ranch.

Eleven years later, Ruth's husband passed away. She mentioned this in her Christmas card to Paul and his wife. After some years, a Christmas letter from Paul informed Ruth that his wife was suffering from Alzheimer's. Not knowing the extent of his wife's illness, Ruth sent him an article describing a blue algae reported as helpful in alleviating Alzheimer's. When Paul phoned to thank her, she invited him to her ranch, more than 200 miles from his home.

"Would it really be all right?" asked Paul, ever considerate. "What will the neighbors think?"

"I don't have any neighbors," laughed Ruth, knowing how isolated her property was.

So Paul accepted her invitation, and they had a delightful, very proper visit.

They had not seen each other for 17 years, but their friendship was easily renewed. Paul really enjoyed Ruth's pot roast and apple pie. "She's a really good cook," he told me.

* There certainly must have been a strong tie from the past for Paul to travel 200 miles to see Ruth again. And what a treat it was to have Ruth's companionship and a home-cooked meal after so many lonely years of caring for a wife degenerating from Alzheimer's disease.

HOW WERE YOU ATTRACTED TO EACH OTHER?

Ruth recalls her impression of Paul when, many years ago, he came into her office at the defense company. He was cheerful and radiant, with a twinkle in his eye, and had a sense of humor. "If someone in the office went to the counter to help Paul before I could, I was disappointed." Thus, she liked him from the start.

Paul also remembers Ruth from those days. "She was vivacious and pleasant to work with; a genuine, outgoing personality."

Both Ruth and Paul were, and still are confident, extroverted personalities and appreciate these traits in each other. Though their lives went in different directions for many years, their mutual attraction remained, leading to the thought that both of them expressed: "It was nice to renew our friendship again."

HOW DID YOUR RELATIONSHIP DEVELOP?

Paul was happy and excited about reconnecting with Ruth. However, he thought he should not contact her right away because, "she'd think I was too anxious." About a month later he phoned her, and again the next month. At that stage it was just "friendship" calls. Ruth enjoyed talking with him but, although she liked him a lot, she had made up her mind she would *not* get married again.

Paul had been taking care of his wife for 10 years. She was showing an increasingly vegetative state, and it had been a long time since he had had any real companionship. As he said, "When I saw Ruth so full of life and vigor, I realized how nice it would be to have that kind of partnership again."

* My heart goes out to the families of those suffering from Alzheimer's disease. What a loss that is of the person you used to know and love. My mother had Alzheimer's, and before she died she didn't know who I was or even who she was. It brought home to me graphically how much our sense of identity is made up of memories. When we lose those memories, we lose the sense of who we are and

> who our dear ones are. Thus Paul had already lost his wife long before he became involved with Ruth.

Paul had sold his building supply company and, as part of his responsibility in his recent position as director of sales for a larger but similar company, he had opportunities to inspect meeting facilities around the country. This meant that local hotels (or a city Chamber of Commerce) would provide complimentary travel, rooms, and meals as they displayed their services to people like Paul. An opportunity for such a trip became available, and he asked Ruth to accompany him. At first, she was uncertain about going with him, but she had friends in the city to which they would travel, and she could stay with them. She called Paul, telling him she would go and that she would make her own arrangements. Then very soon she received an airline ticket and the hotel brochure showing a picture of a luxurious guest room with a king-size bed! "What a presumptuous rascal!" she thought.

Then she had second thoughts: "I'm 71 and he is 73 years old. Why should I be such a prude?" She went with him and had a wonderful time. Twenty-five couples attended from all over the country and participated in many enjoyable activities. Oh yes, she also visited her friends but stayed in the hotel with Paul, becoming sexually involved. A photo in their home, taken during this first trip together, showed the two of them looking glowing and jubilant.

After this first trip, they visited frequently, meeting at Paul's home in a distant city and in Ruth's rural area. Considering what their children would think and their own religious ethics, they agreed not to live together without marrying. Because Paul's wife was still alive, it would be necessary for him to obtain a divorce. This is not an infrequent practice in such situations. His lawyer prepared the legal papers for the divorce, which included the stipulation that he would continue to financially support his debilitated wife until her death. He did so until she died, six years after he and Ruth were married.

After the divorce was official, they were married at the church in Ruth's rural community, followed by a reception at her home. Their country road was lined with pink balloons and directional signs so their 150 guests could find the way to the ranch. All their children and close friends came, happily accepting this new relationship. They honeymooned in Bermuda. As Paul and Ruth talked about the wedding and their happy memories, I could see a glow on both of their animated faces.

For the first five years of their marriage, they maintained Paul's house, since once a month they traveled to that area, each time visiting Paul's wife in a nursing home. Realizing the cost of maintaining his home, Paul decided to sell. His children took over the task of regularly visiting their mother, even though she no longer recognized them. After a five-year transition period, Paul found that he could close out 42 years of his previous life and not miss it. He had made a new life with Ruth.

WHAT WERE YOUR PREVIOUS RELATIONSHIPS LIKE?

Both Ruth and Paul had happy first marriages that ended with long periods of caretaking.

Ruth

Ruth was married at age 18 to her 25-year-old husband. He was a machinist, working all his career in a military defense company. It was a good and loving marriage.

They had one daughter. Ruth's husband contracted emphysema about 20 years into their marriage, and for his benefit, they decided to leave the city to get out of the smog. They purchased their ranch in 1970, and her husband then retired at age 57. For two years they worked at renovating the ranch and moved there in 1972. The cleaner air made Ruth's husband feel much better at first, but gradually his condition deteriorated. Within four years of the move, his activities were limited. By 1978 he was bedridden. In addition to emphysema, he had severe back problems and was hospitalized for three months after back surgery. He was on strong pain pills and oxygen before he died in 1981 of congestive heart failure. Ruth and he knew he was dying, and they had time to cry together and say goodbye.

For five difficult years Ruth took care of her husband, including such nursing duties as bathing him and giving medication, She took care of all the household duties plus all the work on the ranch. She tended the horses, cattle, ducks, and worked in the gardens. It was exhausting, and yet for Ruth, the work on the ranch and in the gardens helped her to keep her balance. One way she took care of herself was to take every Wednesday afternoon off to meet with a quilting group.

Understandably, her husband became more and more irritable as his illness progressed. Ruth still regrets once saying, "If you were this crabby when we first knew each other, I never would have married you."

"Words are like bullets shot from a gun. Once out, you can't take them back," she told me with tears in her eyes.

* Here I think Ruth is being hard on herself. Caring for a seriously ill loved one is extremely wearing, emotionally and physically, and it is very difficult to be continually patient.

Like Ruth's husband, my late husband became irritable when in pain, and there were times when I lost my temper. I regret those times, but I do forgive myself, as I hope Ruth forgives herself.

After her husband's death, Ruth continued living alone on the ranch for more than nine years before she and Paul became romantically involved. At first, the loss of her husband felt like a loss of part of herself. Gradually, life began to be good again as she attended clubs, saw women friends, and gave dinner parties, as Ruth loves to cook. "But," said Ruth, "Never in my wildest dreams did I expect to be as happy again as I am now in my new life with Paul. It is possible to love a second time."

* I very much identify with Ruth, although my caretaking lasted only three months, while Ruth's was for more than five years. During those last few months, my late husband's cancer spread to his internal organs, and he was admitted to a hospice program so that he could die at home. Like Ruth and her husband, we had time to review our life together and to say goodbye. I was able to take off from work to be his prime caretaker. Hospice provided a part-time aide so that I could grocery shop and even see a few clients. Despite this help, care for my husband consumed me.

As Ruth held on to a part of herself by working on the ranch, my work as a psychotherapist was a saving grace. Certainly I never imagined then, nor in the years of grief after my husband's death, that, as did Ruth, I would one day find myself in a joyful life with a new love.

Paul

Paul had married at age 20, while still in college. His wife, one year older, was a good wife and mother to their three children. They have now provided Paul with nine grandchildren and six great grandchildren.

When Paul was 62 years old, his wife first began to exhibit symptoms of Alzheimer's disease. "She often traveled with me when I was working. Then one evening she couldn't find our room in a hotel. Another time she couldn't find her way home from the local beauty shop. Soon I had to take her car keys away and drive her everywhere."

Paul hired a live-in maid who served as a caretaker while he worked. His wife remained at home for nine years before he had to place her in a care facility. During these years she continued to deteriorate. "I'd arrive home from work, and she'd look at me and say, 'When are you taking me home?' She didn't know who I was or who she was." Paul was visibly upset as he continued, "Life was closing in for me. I had only my work and my concern for my wife. I never knew from day to day what crisis would be next. She became belligerent and one time threw an iron at the maid, whom I had to take to the hospital for stitches."

None of Paul's three children lived nearby, so they had difficulty believing how badly their mother had deteriorated. Finally a daughter and then a son took her to their homes for a period of time and gained a better understanding of the problem. The children gave their parents a 50th anniversary party when their mother was in the nursing home. She recognized no one at the party.

Paul went on, "My work and the traveling it entailed helped me to keep my sanity. It was an escape for me, and I still feel guilty about it."

* I hope Paul doesn't feel too guilty. Just as Ruth needed her ranch chores, he needed his work to keep the concern for his wife from consuming him completely.

I know from personal experience that simply putting an Alzheimer patient in a nursing home does not remove the emotional burden. After I placed my mother in a home in which she had good care, I received almost daily

> phone calls. She refused to take baths. She tried to run away. And so it went until her death.

Paul put his arm around Ruth and told me, "We both hold on to fond memories of our departed mates. And it is easy for us to share these memories with each other."

Ruth responded, "We are both mature and have no jealousy about our past relationships."

Paul added, "That's true. And we thank God every day for the happiness we have found in our love for each other."

WHAT ARE YOUR ON-GOING LIVES LIKE?

Ruth and Paul described very few problems in their relationship. One adjustment that they did make is described in Chapter 21, *Monetary and Legal Arrangements.* Certainly they represent a happy, well-adjusted couple who married in later years. I observed this when they interacted together warmly, recalling happy memories and going through a picture album of foreign travel. They have 30 collections of photographs from such places as Australia, New Zealand, the Caribbean, Hong Kong, Thailand, and countries in Europe. Said Paul, "We won't stop traveling until we have to."

> * They are fortunate. Not all older couples have the financial ability or good enough health to travel so extensively.

They cooperate on many household chores. While Ruth does the cooking, Paul sets the table. He dries the dishes as Ruth washes them. Paul helps Ruth with house cleaning, and they enjoy making their bed together. They like sharing work in their gardens. Ruth wants Paul to look nice, so she spends time ironing his shirts, although he believes this is unnecessary.

Television is not important to them, but they do watch the news and some public broadcast programs. Paul likes to read mystery novels. Ruth continues her hobby of making quilts and meets weekly with a group of women engaged in this activity.

As our discussion concluded, Ruth thoughtfully said, "At this point in life, we don't have to face the problems we had in our young marriages. Then there were so many things that were new to us. Now we know what's required, and things go along more smoothly. Life is easier and we have fun."

FINAL THOUGHTS

Ruth and Paul are an example of two mature, loving individuals who devotedly cared for seriously ill spouses for many years. When a person is in the midst of such an experience, it can be all consuming. Often there is little else left of life except perhaps necessary work, in or out of the home. Such work often can be a godsend, as it is one way to hold on to an integral part of one's self.

Years of caretaking provide time to gradually say goodbye to a loved one. During this process, it is very difficult to imagine that you will ever love again, or indeed, ever be truly happy again. But Ruth and Paul did find love and joy in their new life together, and their difficult past experiences have made this happiness even more precious.

Chapter 3

(Interview: Naomi and David)

HEALTH CHANGES WITH TIME; AFFECTION LASTS

"There are days when I'm so sorry I got into this relationship, because I can't paint, I can't do this, I can't do that … and there are other days when I say thank God I've got him!"

THEME
Entering the Caretaker Role

Although David is just three years older than Naomi, his health and memory have deteriorated in the past few years. Naomi's straightforward, honest approach in talking with me was instructive and enlightening. Her advice to women readers, based on her experience is, "If you marry an older man, you're going to be a nurse." But there is no lack of love in her honesty.

INTRODUCING NAOMI AND DAVID

Naomi was 64 when they met; David was 67. Now she's 78 and he's 81. Naomi had been widowed since she was 46, more than 18 years, when she met David, whose wife had died a few months earlier.

With this couple, it is interesting to follow the changes over time; 14 years of being together, with 13 years of marriage.

David and Naomi live in a large retirement community. As I entered the apartment, the mezuzah on the door clearly identified their Judaism. Inside the sunny, spacious apartment were many paintings of Jewish life, including the Torah, the Sabbath candles, and a rabbi, all painted by Naomi. She is an intelligent, energetic woman who talks and laughs easily and is pleasant to look at. She is somewhat tall with short, curly gray hair. David is a friendly, cheerful man of medium height, slightly built, and neatly dressed in a tan shirt and matching tan slacks.

HOW DID YOU MEET?

They were living in the same city; David in his large family home, and Naomi in an apartment. She sold her house 10 years after her husband's death. One evening, Naomi's friend invited her to their synagogue to hear a woman rabbi preside, while David was there to say prayers for his recently deceased wife. When they met, he asked Naomi to go to dinner after the service. She declined, as she and her friend had planned to go out to dinner, but she gave him her phone number.

David called her that night and was at her house by 9:00 the next morning! He wore shorts and, as Naomi said with a smile, "He looked adorable." They ate dinner out that night and later danced in her apartment. They have seen each other every day since.

> ✻ David certainly wasted no time in connecting with Naomi! His wife had been dead a few months, and I believe that for David, it was very difficult to be alone.
>
> Men tend not to have the same social and support circle as do women, and so often a man's wife is his only in-

timate friend. Often little boys are socialized not to express feelings, so often it is difficult for men to allow themselves much time to grieve. Both of these factors lead to finding a new partner fairly soon after a wife's death, often to avoid loneliness and grief. David, particularly, had a great need to be loved and cared for, and his early years, which I'll describe soon, made his needs particularly strong.

HOW WERE YOU ATTRACTED TO EACH OTHER?

After the many years of being alone, Naomi was finally ready for an intimate relationship. "David was attractive and fun. I didn't want a great intellectual; I've had enough of that. He's very likable. He likes the whole world. I'm very happy. There are days I'd like to break his neck, but that has nothing do with it. He's very right for me at this stage of my life." I then asked Naomi, why not at an earlier stage? "If we were raising children, he would love the kids to pieces but wouldn't push them enough intellectually." Finally, David 's being Jewish and involved in the temple were very important to her.

What attracted David to Naomi? He liked her hair, her body, the way she looked and dressed. "She was different, full of pep and smiling. I liked the way she moved her hands during that first service when I saw her. It was like leading an orchestra, and she still does it!"

* David is a somewhat passive man, and it is understandable that he would be attracted to Naomi's vivaciousness.

HOW DID YOUR RELATIONSHIP DEVELOP?

After David and Naomi met, they spent a great deal of time together, sharing ideas and life stories. "Do you remember, David," said Naomi, "that restaurant where someone came over and asked if we were newlyweds? We couldn't stop talking to each other. This went on for hours and hours," she laughed. "It was crazy — we really couldn't stop. We finally reached a point where we could be quiet occasionally."

They became sexually involved after several weeks, both having been celibate for a long time. "His erections came slowly, but they worked," confided Naomi, "and, like the talking, we couldn't stop!"

According to Naomi, David was nervous about being sexually involved outside of marriage and was sure the neighbors saw him coming and going from her apartment. He decided they had to get married. Naomi had some doubts, particularly as to whether David's daughters would accept her, but she cared for David very much and was tired of living alone. So, married they were.

Because Jewish law decrees not marrying for a year after a spouse's death, they were first married by a judge in Naomi's apartment seven months after they met. Naomi recalled that it was late January because it was the day of the Superbowl game, and the judge was late because he had been watching it. The guests didn't mind since they also had a good time watching the game before the wedding. A Jewish wedding in the temple was held in March.

After they were married, David sold his house and moved into Naomi's apartment. He appears to have had no difficulty with this decision, as his big house was difficult for him to maintain, and he just didn't want to be by himself. After six years, they found a new home, moving into the retirement community where they have lived for eight years.

* For a couple, finding and furnishing a new home together gives a truly satisfactory sense of belonging. It becomes *their* home instead of *his or her* home.

WHAT WERE YOUR EARLY LIVES LIKE?

David and Naomi both had difficult backgrounds.

David

David was raised from infancy in an Orthodox Jewish orphanage after his parents were killed in an automobile accident. He had four siblings, whom in later life he tried to locate by every means possible, but with no success.

In the orphanage he learned Hebrew, leading eventually to his becoming a teacher in a yeshiva. He left the orphanage at age 15 and joined the Civilian Conservation Corps (a government agency created in the Depression of the 1930s to provide labor-type work for the unemployed). He was on his own until he married at 35. He worked his way through college as a truck driver.

Naomi

When Naomi was four, her parents divorced. She and her older brother grew up in a Jewish neighborhood where divorce was unheard of. Being thoroughly ashamed, she lied and said that her father was dead. Her mother worked in the garment industry and was very involved with the union. Explained Naomi, "My brother and I were an after thought with her. She was there for us, but we weren't the big thing in her life. The big thing in her life was the world." Her mother wouldn't let her father visit when she was a child, but as an adult, she found him and stayed in touch until his death at age 99.

> * With her mother's work and involvement in her trade union, and her father's absence, Naomi grew up very much on her own. I believe this has a good deal to do with her

being the strong woman she is today. I have worked with many women who were strong on the outside but had an inner core that longed for the love and affection they lacked in childhood. I believe this is true of Naomi. David, raised in an orphanage with a great unmet need for family, is insecure because of the intensity of this need.

Despite difficult and lonely times in their early years, both Naomi and David were strong enough to make good lives for themselves, and to give each other the affection and attention that was lacking in their childhoods.

WHAT WERE YOUR PREVIOUS RELATIONSHIPS LIKE?

David

When David married, he was working as a teacher in a yeshiva. His first wife, Esther, had a 16-year-old daughter from a previous marriage, and they also had a daughter together. David noted, "Naomi takes care of me as I took care of Esther. I did all the shopping and paid the bills."

* As a younger, healthier man, David was the caretaker. Now Naomi, as the caretaker, is very much in charge but finds the increased responsibility difficult. David must feel a loss of pride and control as he becomes more dependent. The gradual deterioration of health and memory changes the balance of power in a relationship and presents problems for both the caregiver and the care receiver.

David's wife was not well for many years, and during the interview he was confused as to the cause of her ill health and death. Naomi told me that Esther suffered from hepatitis that became worse until she died of liver failure. Their sex life was infrequent because of Esther's health, yet David remained faithful. It was an affectionate marriage, and he still misses her. There were tears in his eyes as he talked about her, although he does not share these feelings with Naomi. If Naomi talks of her deceased husband, he gets angry and leaves the room.

> ✻ David is jealous of Naomi's late husband. To feel some jealousy is normal, but to act on this jealousy by walking out of the room closes the door literally and figuratively on Naomi's sharing this part of her life with him. This limits the free exchange and closeness between them.
>
> I too, feel some jealousy when Jerry talks of his late wife, but I know she was a part of his life for 45 years. It would be almost impossible for him to talk about his past life without mentioning her, just as I cannot talk about my past without mentioning my husband of 35 years. Jerry also admits to some jealousy.
>
> Though a certain amount of discomfort is to be expected, there cannot be genuine sharing if you must avoid a huge chunk of your life. In fantasy, I would like to be the only person Jerry had ever loved, but it's just that—a fantasy. At one time or another, we all may have had similar fantasies, but we need to accept the reality of past relationships. The past is part of each of us, and we need to bring our whole self into a new relationship.

Naomi

Naomi was wedded to her first husband for 26 years. They married when they were both 21 and had just graduated from college.

He worked as an architect, and they moved frequently throughout the United States, while she was a housewife, raising their two daughters. During this time she had a studio and painted. She describes this marriage as "better than most." Her husband died suddenly of a heart attack, making it particularly difficult for Naomi to accept the reality of his death. "I expected him home at any time," she reminisced.

> * This reaction is not at all unusual. Often after the death of a spouse, especially when there has been a long marriage, the survivor can sense the presence of the deceased. A wife may frequently turn around to talk to a husband who is no longer there. For quite a few years after his death, I often found myself thinking thoughts in the very same words that my late husband used.
>
> When two people are close, they take in parts of each other. Now I sometimes hear Jerry's voice when I'm thinking, so gradually he is becoming part of me.

Some time after her husband's death, Naomi, having gone directly from her mother's home into her long marriage, "found being on my own to be one of the most exciting things that had ever happened to me." She worked as a manager for an art gallery. She dated frequently but didn't want any commitments.

> * Working did a great deal for Naomi's self-esteem and helped her to deal with her grief. **Karin**, also widowed after a long marriage, found work that helped her to develop more fully as an independent person. Many of the women I have known in counseling, especially if they had spent many years as homemakers, gained a great deal of confidence by performing well on a job.

My work as a therapist was so engrossing that in the early stages of grief, after my first husband's death, the sessions spent with clients were the only times I felt completely myself again. Working at a satisfying job is a good antidote to grief and a boost to self-esteem because it gives pleasure in accomplishment and pride in newly found abilities.

WHAT ADJUSTMENTS HAVE YOU MADE IN YOUR RELATIONSHIP?

Naomi had been widowed and on her own for 18 years, while David had lived for 32 years with his first wife. To quote Naomi, "Living with another person, no matter whom, can be difficult. Especially for someone like me who's been alone so many years. It took me 10 years with David to say *we* instead of *me*."

Naomi had to adjust to David's jealousy of other men. "He's jealous and insecure, but this behavior has gotten easier to live with." When we discussed this issue together, David said there were two men they saw at temple gatherings who paid a lot of attention to Naomi and whom he thought she liked. Naomi joked and laughed with her New York accent, "Just one. There was another one, but I dropped him. I don't even talk to him now when I see him—no big deal." She adjusted by giving David less cause for jealousy.

* Naomi softens the dilemma of David's jealousy with humor by saying, "I dropped him—no big deal." She protects David from the pain of his suspicions and herself from any possible accusations. To accept a partner's even casual friendship with members of the opposite sex, an individual must be secure in his or her own self-worth. David's childhood, with no loving family, did not lead to

> a strong internal sense of security. His declining health increased his need for Naomi, thus most likely his fear of losing her, and in turn, his jealousy. With humor and some restriction of her own gregariousness, Naomi has decreased the conflict around this issue.

David made a lot of adjustments to please Naomi. He stopped his use of profanity, and she got him to take his hat off in the house. In view of David's upbringing in an orphanage, it is clear why Naomi had to "civilize" him. In many ways, Naomi is in charge of this relationship.

WHAT ARE YOUR ON-GOING ACTIVITIES"

For recreation and entertainment, the balance of power seems equal. David and Naomi make mutual decisions about recreation and social activities. They go to musical comedies together and enjoy old-time records and classical music. Naomi taught David to play Scrabble, while he taught her card games, and they share these games with friends. She plays table tennis with a group of women, and while she does this, David plays pool with the husbands.

Until recently David had been an enthusiastic golfer and fisherman. He has had to stop temporarily because of ill health. Naomi has a college degree in art and has never stopped painting and taking art classes. She is quite talented and works in various media. At the end of my visit, I had the pleasure of seeing her studio and viewing the many paintings there. At present she attends a regular weekly art group at the retirement community. This is one separate activity that Naomi finds important enough to continue despite the increasing need to spend more time with David. David accepts this absence. This shows a flexibility in their relationship and a respect for separate interests.

MOVING TOWARD THE CARETAKER ROLE

David's health and short-term memory have been declining over the past number of years. An MRI (Magnetic Resonance Imaging diagnosis) was taken recently, and calcification in the brain was diagnosed. Sometimes David forgets what Naomi said five minutes after she says it. As I was leaving, David asked me to go out to dinner with them and I politely declined his offer since I had another appointment. He went on to ask me at least three more times as if he had never heard my answer. Naomi reminded David of my appointment and this was helpful to him. When we discussed his forgetfulness, David was in denial.

* It is frightening to start to lose your memory, and David pretends to himself that it isn't happening. Naomi is very aware of the problem and helps David when his short-term memory fails him. By helping her husband in this way, she is gracefully adjusting to the caretaker role.

Seven years ago David had a triple bypass operation and also a gall bladder operation. Shortly before my visit, he had several incidents of fainting for an unknown reason. The doctor suspected that his blood-pressure medication was too strong and lowered it. The incidents were so recent that David is not driving, golfing, or fishing, for fear that he might faint again. He must stay home a great deal and wants Naomi to stay with him. She told me frankly that she resents this, as it keeps her from so much that she wants to do.

* Naomi's admission and acceptance of this resentment is healthy. Too many spouses secretly think this way and feel guilty. By hiding their resentment, even from themselves, it might leak out in sarcasm or irritability.

> To resent is not to stop loving or to stop doing what is necessary to care for your ailing mate. My deceased husband, even before he suffered from cancer, had numerous hospitalizations for phlebitis (clotting of blood in his legs). Many of the things we enjoyed together we could no longer do. I believe I took good care of him until the end, but inside of me, in addition to the adult love and sadness, was an angry little child who wanted to have fun and to be cared for, and it was I who had to take care of him. In accepting this childlike part of myself, it made me more capable of functioning as a loving caretaker.

Despite her difficulty with the caretaker role, Naomi expresses her satisfaction with the marriage. "David's one of the sweetest guys you'll ever meet. Every day he tells me over and over 'I love you.' There's lots of physical affection, hugs and kisses, cuddling in bed. I think the average woman wants what I've got. I know he loves me. I've never doubted that for an instant."

FINAL THOUGHTS

At this point in their lives, Naomi and David are a good fit. Naomi is strong and takes care of David. Understandably, he somewhat resents Naomi's bossiness. But for the first time in his life, he's being nurtured, and in return, he gives Naomi the love and adoration she so much appreciates. This love and affection compensates Naomi for giving up so many activities that have been important to her so that she can care for David.

I know, as do David and Naomi, that as the health of one partner changes with time, feelings of resentment in the caretaker are not sinful and that love and affection can last.

Chapter 4

(Interview: Nancy and Pat)

COMMITTED TRUE LOVE ... LIVING SEPARATELY

When Nancy and Pat first became involved, they remained in their own homes, visiting each other regularly. Now they live in separate apartments in a retirement community. They have never considered marriage or living together, and this suits their different lifestyles. They have both their closeness and some private time. They like the arrangement this way.

THEME
Late-Life Liberation

Both Nancy and Pat come from long, stable, conventional marriages, devoted to the raising of children. Now Nancy is delighted to be more than a cookie-baking grandmother. Their separate living arrangements makes for mutual joy when they reunite. As noted by Nancy, "Each time I see Pat after a few days of no contact, I experience the anticipation of going on a very special date."

With no children to raise or jobs to tie them down, they add zest to their lives by traveling extensively. Now in their later years, they experience more freedom and adventure than ever before.

INTRODUCING NANCY AND PAT

Nancy is 75 years old. Pat is nearly 77. She has been widowed for 16 years, and Pat's wife died six years ago. They are a very close, committed couple living in separate one-bedroom, one-bath apartments located about a mile apart. Both are Catholic, and particularly for Nancy, religion is very important.

I first visited Nancy in her apartment where she has been living for only six weeks. It was as neat as a pin and pleasantly furnished with traditional pieces. Pictures of her children and grandchildren were displayed, and the refrigerator door had photos of Nancy and Pat together. I was particularly attracted by a photo of Nancy and Pat on a hiking trail, Pat with a wooden staff in one hand, and his other arm around Nancy. They looked happy. He appeared very Irish, with a square jaw and intense eyes.

Nancy is a tall, attractive woman with curly, graying hair. She greeted me warmly, and we sat at her dining room table to talk. Nancy has a way of making fun of herself. She waves her hands, and in a high-pitched voice laughingly talks about her children, who expect her to be "a good little mother and grandmother." I asked her if she's saying that her role for years was the good, sweet, all-giving Catholic mother and that she is intimating, "I'm a different woman now." Nancy agreed. Actually, Nancy is still a good Catholic and a loving mother and grandmother, but her relationship with Pat has freed her to be, in many ways, a more liberated woman.

After conducting the interview with Nancy, I drove a mile to Pat's apartment. The layout of the two apartments was identical, but they couldn't have looked more different. Pat's place was very cluttered, and the furniture was older and simpler. One entire wall was lined with books. In front of the couch was a large television set. Pat sat on the couch as we talked. He was casually dressed in shorts and a red T-shirt, with somewhat of a belly exposed beneath the shirt. He laughed frequently and heartily as we talked.

HOW DID YOU MEET?

Nancy and Pat have known each other for 45 years. They both came to live in the same suburban area as newlyweds. In the course of Nancy's marriage, she had two children, while Pat and his wife had seven. They joined the same Catholic church, and gradually Nancy and Pat's wife, Amanda, became friends, carpooling to take their children to the same Catholic school. When Nancy's youngest child was in the third grade, she obtained a position as a sales woman for the local gift shop. Somewhat later she found Amanda a job in the same store. Then in the 1950s, Nancy and Amanda formed an eight-woman support group that lasted 15 years. When at Amanda's home, Nancy would sometimes see Pat, and she also would see him at church and at church functions, although the two couples did not socialize together. To Pat, Nancy was "just a pleasant lady I saw in my wife's women's group."

HOW DID YOUR RELATIONSHIP DEVELOP?

Nancy retired from her job at the gift shop after working there for 22 years. She wanted to write her family history and joined the memoir-writing class that Pat was already attending. By that time, Amanda had come down with breast cancer and was ill for two years before passing away. Nancy had promised her that she would help Pat get to their memoir-writing class. He needed transportation, as he was suffering from macular degeneration and cataracts of the eyes. Nancy also began to drive him to his doctor appointments.

After retiring from her job, Nancy became a hospice volunteer, and in that capacity learned about the stages of grieving. When

Pat asked her to go with him to see a movie, she didn't know what to reply. She told a counselor at the hospice, "I just don't think he's grieving right." The counselor replied, "Just be a friend." So she accepted Pat's invitation. That's when their relationship started to become more of a genuine friendship, about three months after Amanda's death.

Pat and Nancy continued going to the writing class together for five years, and they recently finished their memoirs. They had dinner out after class and also went to the movies, seeing each other about twice a week. Gradually they became physically affectionate—holding hands in the movie, exchanging a friendly hug, and kissing goodbye (a little stronger if they'd been separated for a while). About six months after Amanda died, they had sexual relations. To their surprise and delight, their sex life was more free and fulfilling than ever before. "I never in a thousand years believed I was capable of being so open and expressive sexually," Nancy exclaimed.

When they became sexually involved, Nancy and Pat remained in their separate homes where they had raised their families but spent frequent nights together. This suited their different living styles. As Pat said, "I never clutter up her house. She never complains about my mess, although she did make me clean up my bathroom." Although Pat once told Nancy, "If you want to get married, we'll get married." Nancy thought marriage would constrain her from leading her own life and spending her own money as she pleased. She and Pat have committed themselves to always being together and to taking care of each other if either becomes ill or disabled. That seems sufficient to them.

With the completion of her family memoirs, Nancy felt a letdown. The winter rains came, and the house in which she had lived for 38 years felt too big. Pat also had a large house with stairs he had difficulty climbing and which required extensive upkeep. They had visited friends in an apartment with the same layout as their present two apartments and in the same retirement community where they now live. They both agreed that the retirement community would better suit their needs.

Both of their homes sold quickly, and because their present apartments cost less than they had gained from the sale of their houses, they ended up with a financial gain. When I visited them, they were both recently established in their new homes. They each needed to dispose of much of their furniture before moving into their small apartments. I asked Nancy if the move from her home where she had lived for so many years, and the disposing of so many possessions, was sorrowful for her. She said it wasn't.

> * One factor that made their move much easier was that their children divided their furniture between them. Thus, they each knew that they would see their precious possessions again when they visited their children. The same held true for **Leonard** when he moved to **Barbara's** country home. His children also divided up his furniture, making his move much easier for him emotionally.

WHAT WERE YOUR EARLY LIVES LIKE?

Nancy

Nancy grew up in a small community during the Depression. Her father was manager of a laundry. She had "a good, simple life." Her parents were affectionate, and she had two much-older aunts who lived nearby and were loving toward her, although they were strict. Both of her parents are now dead, but she has one brother who lives at a distance. He has met Pat and gets along well with him.

* Nancy's stable, happy childhood has led to her being a sensible, secure, affectionate woman, capable of forming such a good relationship with Pat. Her being raised in the '30s and '40s, when a woman's role was very limited, led to her being "a good little mother and grandmother," as she would laughingly refer to herself. While she is still a good mother and grandmother, she has the independence of mind to fashion a relationship with Pat very different from the conventional expectations of the age in which she was raised.

Pat

Pat was the eldest of three children. His father worked as a sales manager for a large company after retiring from the military. In both capacities, the family moved frequently. Though his brother became very social, Pat had more difficulty making friends with the family's frequent moves, relying more on his own company and his love of books. He was close to and admired his father, but was distant from his mother, whom he described as "a chronic hypochondriac." As he says, "She always thought she was going to die of something." His mother came from a wealthy family, and the children were raised mostly by a housekeeper. Before the birth of his younger sister, when he was 10 years old, Pat was told only that his mother was going to be ill for a long time. Subsequently, he was left with his maternal grandparents for a year. They paid little attention to him, and he took care of himself by reading from their extensive library.

As a young man, Pat had two years of college and then entered the army during World War II. When discharged, he traveled across the country, ending up on the West Coast. He held many different jobs, most of them in sales. His mother was disappointed that he did not become a professional, since his brother had earned a Ph.D. Both of his parents are now deceased, and his brother and sister are living in other states. Nancy has met them both, and she and Pat have traveled with Pat's brother. Both of Pat's siblings have accepted his relationship with Nancy.

> * Pat's frequent moves as a child led him to form a great deal of reliance on his own inner strength. He became independent and adventurous, moving west, and defying family expectations in finding work that suited him. He brings this sense of adventure into his relationship with Nancy. In her he has found the loving, affectionate woman that he lacked in his mother.

THEIR LONG, STABLE MARRIAGES

Nancy

Nancy was married at age 23, at which time she moved out of her parents' home, never having the experience of living independently. This was the norm for women of her time. Her husband was an accountant and made a good living. He was reliable and responsible, taking good care of Nancy and their three children. She did not work until her youngest child was in the third grade. Her husband was more introverted and much less adventurous that Pat is. When Nancy thinks of some of the challenging experiences Pat had with his young family, she believes she would have been apprehensive of such ventures with her children. Also, her husband offered her much more financial stability than Pat could have, so Pat might not have been as right for her at this earlier stage of her life.

On the negative side, Nancy has mentioned that her husband was a worrier and "master of the put-down." True to her role as a good wife, Nancy did not fight back, and the marriage was fairly conflict free.

> * When resentment is held in and not expressed, this often leads to a lack of affection, spontaneity, and joy. When I look back on my first marriage, I realize that there were times when my annoyed tone of voice, while speaking to my husband, was in effect, a put-down of him. He said nothing, and I believe now this resulted in less affection shown to me.
>
> Nancy is careful not to make this mistake with Pat. Because of what she experienced in her marriage, she never puts Pat down for his faults, such as a lack of neatness and organization. This frees them to express more fully their affection and love.

Nancy's husband died of colon cancer. He was ill for two years, and during the last six months they had the support of a hospice service. After his death, hospice offered Nancy comfort during her grieving, as did her women's group. Very important was her continuing to work as a way of keeping her mind active and her body busy.

Pat

After Pat moved to the West Coast, he met his future wife at a Catholic gathering for young people. He was 27, and she was 25 years old. They married a few months later and had seven children. He describes his marriage as a good one. Pat showed me a picture of himself and his wife in his memoirs. They were a handsome couple.

Pat's main conflict with his wife was over financial security. When he worked in sales, they had weeks with no income. Pat told me, " During these periods she thought we were going to die of starvation. I was completely confident we would be all right. Sometimes I'd go six weeks between jobs, and I'd have lots of fun doing all sorts of things, while she got madder and madder." They had arguments about what his wife thought were his extravagances, such as his buying a rifle for a Mountain Man competition. She also worried a great deal about the children. Certainly seven children are a lot to worry about!

* His wife's worrying was perfectly natural, given the circumstances. Pat was rebelling against some of the same negative traits he found in his mother, who, according to him, always thought her children "were about to die any minute." It is not uncommon to unconsciously choose a mate to repeat some of the patterns of childhood.

Now, both Nancy's and Pat's comfortable financial circumstances make for more freedom from monetary concern than during Pat's marriage. Nancy has her own separate income, and Pat can be free to spend on special treats, as he has his retirement income plus a substantial sum from the sale of his family home.

Amanda was seriously ill with breast cancer for two years. When she died, it was "kind of a relief" to Pat because of her suffering. He went off on a trip right after she died, admitting that "I didn't have much of a mourning period." On the trip he camped out and read *Huckleberry Finn.* (Pat could be considered much like Mark Twain's literary character.) He reminisces, "I wanted to do something different to occupy my mind. I really enjoyed myself."

* It is not unusual for someone with a mate who has been ill for a long time to feel relief when death comes. A good deal of the mourning has been done during the illness. I am struck by Pat's ability to find enjoyment being alone, even after the most difficult of circumstances. He might have developed this capacity as a child. In his grandparents' home, he was ignored but he found pleasure in reading, just as he now did after his wife passed away.

WHAT PROBLEMS WERE FACED AND WHAT ADJUSTMENTS WERE MADE?

Nancy and Pat report very few problems, and perhaps their separate living arrangement makes this possible. Certainly, living together would be difficult, with Nancy so neat and Pat so disorganized. When they visit each other, they are able to respect these differences, with Pat not cluttering Nancy's apartment, and Nancy tolerating Pat's mess.

Their respect for each other's differences and their ability to enjoy themselves with or without each other, makes for a smooth relationship. As Pat says, "I don't push her to do what she doesn't want to do, and she doesn't push me. If Nancy doesn't want to engage in an activity with me, I just do it alone, and she does the same."

But still, how can any couple avoid some degree of conflict? Perhaps the answer is that Nancy and Pat don't use the word "conflict." They say they have "heated discussions." An example of one of these discussions is given in Chapter 18, *Personality Differences and Styles of Conflict*, page 218. In reading this, you will see how much their sense of humor and tolerance of each other's styles helped to resolve this disagreement. Nancy knows that Pat is hot tempered, and this doesn't disturb her. Pat appreciates Nancy's ability to calmly resolve the situation. Undoubtedly, they have had many other heated discussions that have been similarly resolved.

WHAT DO YOU VALUE IN EACH OTHER?

Nancy describes Pat as easy going, affectionate, and kind. To her, "He is interesting—an historian, always ready for a new adventure. And, he is a wonderful lover!"

Pat likes Nancy's good nature. He finds her pleasant, never moody or sharp. In the course of our conversation, Pat made enthusiastic statements about Nancy. "How could you not like Nancy?" he said. He showed me his finished memoirs. On the first page of the book, he has a credit "To Nancy, dear critic and editor." When I was talking with both of them together, he said, "I enjoy being with Nancy no matter what we're doing. If we were both in a house fire, I'd enjoy being with Nancy." They both laughed, with Nancy saying, "He'd save me."

WHAT ARE YOUR DAILY AND WEEKLY ROUTINES?

Both Pat and Nancy like the arrangement of living separately and continuing the same routine that they each had in their previous homes. Both value their independent time and spend Monday through Wednesday evenings in their own apartments. Pat likes to watch a movie every night. Nancy washes her hair, writes letters, pays bills, and phones friends. When Thursday arrives, they are both excited and happy to see each other.

They alternate staying at each other's place. In the evening they drink a glass of wine together (they both like *Gewerstermeiner*) and watch the TV news, eating dinner on trays in front of the television. In Nancy's house, she cooks dinner, being careful with salt and fat content, washes the dishes, and makes breakfast the next morning. Pat does the same at his house, usually cooking TV dinners, while Nancy reminds him to make a salad. The one who is visiting gets the first section of the newspaper at breakfast.

Part of their routine is the chore of paying bills. They each have their own expenses. Nancy, being more organized than Pat, handles his bills since previously he had not been paying them on time. He appreciates her help. Nancy also helps Pat keep track of his appointments, as he has begun to have some difficulty with his memory.

> * Memory problems in varying degrees are very common as we grow older. I struggle with memory myself. The name of a person, a book, or a place just vanishes from my mind when I need it but will return later if I relax and don't strain to search for it.
>
> Both Pat and I are absent minded. After interviewing him, I drove him in my car to Nancy's house to talk with the two of them together. Pat put his hiking boots in the back of my car so that he could walk the mile back to his home when we had finished. He asked me to remind him to take the boots out of my car—the blind leading the blind! I completely forgot, and three hours later when stopping en route to my home, I spied the boots. When I phoned Pat, he had forgotten he had left them with me! I mailed them back to him.

WHAT ARE YOUR INTERESTS AND ACTIVITIES?

At home together, they enjoy television, although their tastes are different. Nancy prefers dramatic programs, especially English productions like *Masterpiece Theatre*, while Pat likes Western films.

They compromise and take turns watching both kinds. In movies they also have different tastes. She prefers art films and often goes without Pat to films that only she likes.

* This ability to respect and consider each other's preferences contributes another important factor to the success of this relationship.

Nancy, with a twinkle in her eye, said, "The good thing about having a poor memory is that you can see the same movie twice and enjoy it just as much."

* I find this to be true for me as well—maybe one of the benefits of aging!

Pat has a multitude of hobbies. He grew up with a gun and for years competed as a sharp shooter, attending the Mountain Man competitions. This fit with his love of American history, as evidenced in his bookcase filled with history books, chronologically arranged from the American Revolution to the present. Now he can no longer compete as a sharp shooter because of his eyesight problems. In addition to writing his memoirs, Pat has created an unpublished novel set during the Civil War.

He works in wood and, along with one of his sons, made the attractive redwood-stump table in his living room. When he becomes more established in the retirement community, he plans to join the camera club, the writing club, the hiking club, and to use the woodworking shop.

* True to his enthusiastic nature, perhaps Pat is planning to over-extend himself.

Nancy and Pat every year take two or three trips with their tent trailer. Last year they crossed the country, traveling 7,500 miles. They have been to Hawaii, Alaska, and other places in the U.S., visiting Pat's children or traveling with them. They went to Europe on the anniversary of the Battle of the Bulge during W.W.II, as Pat had been a paratrooper in that battle. When I saw them, they were planning a two-month visit to Italy. Nancy really appreciates traveling with Pat. Her husband used to explode when things went wrong on a trip. In contrast, Pat didn't get upset when the wheel came off of their camper; he merely fixed it. Pat says of traveling with Nancy, "We have fun. She's the person with whom I can do everything I want to do."

FINAL THOUGHTS

Nancy and Pat are a shining example of late-life liberation. Nancy had been a conventional wife and mother but now has the flexibility to maintain a different lifestyle, enjoying a romantic and sexual relationship with a man to whom she is not married. Pat is able to more freely express his adventurous nature now that he has reached the stage of life where he no longer needs to raise and financially support seven children. They have chosen to live separately, and for Nancy and Pat, this gives them the freedom they both desire after their long, duty-filled marriages. Their lifestyles might not be for all older couples newly coupled, but for Nancy and Pat it makes for a happy and deeply committed partnership.

Chapter 5

(Interview Donna and Stuart)

WITH A 26-YEAR AGE DIFFERENCE, CAN THERE BE A SUCCESSFUL UNION?

"He was 78 years old, and I thought I didn't want to get involved with an older man. I wanted someone closer to my age. But no one was around."

"After 56 years with my first wife, I have learned how to handle a woman to keep her loving you. Not a day goes by now that I don't put my arms around Donna a dozen times and tell her how much I love her."

THEME
The Balance of Power in a Very Traditional Marriage

Both Donna and Stuart come from conservative Christian backgrounds. In this loving relationship, their religion defines their roles; the man is the head of the household, and the woman follows his lead. Earlier in their marriage, the 26-year age difference reinforced these roles. Now, as Stuart ages and needs Donna's help, and as Donna grows more self-confident, the balance of power is gradually shifting to a more equal union.

INTRODUCING DONNA AND STUART

Donna is 64 years of age and Stuart is 90. They have been married for 12 years. We sat talking around their dining room table. Donna is a sweet, friendly woman with short gray hair, dressed neatly in pants and a colorful blouse. Stuart is heavy set with a powerful chest and a strong, steady gaze. As we talked, they touched each other and sometimes laughed together.

They live in a house owned by Donna on five acres of land in a rural development. It is nestled among tall oak trees with a rolling lawn leading down to a picturesque abandoned barn. The porch is full of flowerpots and bird feeders. Near the barn is a deer feeding station filled with corn. At night, with the help of a bright porch light, Stuart and Donna can see as many as 10 deer feeding. They both love animals, but the feeder keeps the deer away from the house, where they would eat the roses. Donna told me that once a bear came to the front of the house at three o'clock in the afternoon but went to the deer feeder, spending about 50 minutes eating. The two of them enjoyed watching from behind the safety of their living room window.

Their home contains many pieces of fine, antique furniture that Stuart brought from his house to supplement Donna's furnishings. Rooms are crowded with furniture and numerous knickknacks. On the walls are many plaques with religious sayings.

HOW DID YOU MEET?

Donna has been a part-time volunteer at the local history center for some years. She particularly enjoys taking elementary school students through the attractive exhibits and dramatically telling stories about people and events during the early years. Ordinarily somewhat shy and reserved, she feels free to fully express herself with children. One display is a small working model that shows how gold was extracted from ore in the region and refined. The mechanism is quite old and often has malfunctioned. After a serious breakdown, Donna wanted to find someone who could volunteer to overhaul the machinery.

After asking a friend, she was told that Stuart, living in a nearby small community, might have the skills and equipment to do the job. She contacted him. Yes, he would look at the equipment, but he needed to have the model taken to his house because he was caring for his terminally ill wife. This was done, and after a time, Stuart got the parts operating properly. The exhibit was reinstalled at the history center and worked satisfactorily for a while. But one part broke down again. With Stuart's directions, Donna removed the part and took it to Stuart's house for repair.

Then one day, Stuart phoned Donna to tell her that his wife had passed away. She expressed her sympathy. Thereafter, feeling lonely, Stuart frequently called her and they talked.

HOW WERE YOU ATTRACTED TO EACH OTHER?

Donna saw Stuart as a good Christian, a unique man. He did not use bad language, nor did he have smoking or drinking habits. His extensive traveling in his profession made him fascinating to be with.

Stuart liked Donna's enthusiasm about the merits of the history center and when visiting there, he observed her dramatic performance with the students. "She can be so outgoing and lively, but also so soft and gentle," he remarked. Stuart then noted her physical attractiveness, her sensitivity, and her high sense of values.

HOW DID YOUR RELATIONSHIP DEVELOP?

After Stuart had phoned her a few times, Donna remembered that she had seen an extensive collection of California historical books in his house. Feeling lonely herself, she started visiting with him frequently and with Stuart, looked through his books. Both of them enjoyed this togetherness, and little by little their relationship grew. As Donna said, "Just from his conversation, I could tell where it was going. He was getting serious."

During one visit, Stuart showed Donna a full-length mink cape he still had from his first wife. She put it on, admiring it in a mirror, saying, "I feel elegant." Stuart replied, "You look elegant. If we were of the same religious persuasion, I would ask you to be my wife." His saying this just two months after his wife's death seemed too soon for Donna. They continued seeing each other, visiting each other's homes, having dinners together, and going to services at each other's churches. Then one evening, while in his home, she remarked, "It's so nice to have someone to come home to." Stuart then came over to her, giving her a hug and a first kiss. From then on, they dated more often and Stuart talked about marriage. They each strongly believed that there should be no sexual activity between them until marriage.

As their relationship developed, Donna had some mixed thoughts. "I wanted to marry him, but on the other hand, because of our age difference (she was 52 and he was 78), I didn't want to get involved with an older man again. There had been an age difference of 34 years between my first husband and me. I preferred someone close to my own age, but there was no such man around. Nor did I want a divorced man or one never having been married because I would have to take on his problems, or he might be so set in his ways and habits as to be unwilling to change."

* Of course, a previously married man might also be unwilling to change, but this was Donna's perception.

Another realistic matter important to Donna (and recognized by Stuart), was the fact that she had recently been laid off from her part-time secretarial position, and with no income, her savings were about gone. So they decided to be married. Some friends thought this was too fast since the wedding would take place only 10 months after Stuart's wife had passed away, following his 7 years of caring for her.

> * Many people do not understand that years of caring for an ill spouse are years when the need for love and companionship are not being fulfilled. Also, during an illness there is ample time for preliminary grieving and preparing for the loss so that there need not be a period of time set by convention for a new relationship to start.

The wedding ceremony took place in a private chapel in Las Vegas. They then honeymooned in Hawaii. Donna, who has a delightful sense of humor, told me the following story about their wedding. She had prepared their vows and a tape recording of a friend playing the organ and singing "*Where Thou Goest I Will Go.*" A young couple with a nine-month-old baby, who had just been married in the chapel, were witnesses to their wedding. The ceremony was interrupted periodically by the baby's cries, which together with the playing of Donna's recording, resulted in a longer period than was standard for a Las Vegas wedding. During this time the chapel photographer kept popping in and out, looking at his watch. But the vows and the music went as planned and despite the interruptions, Donna and Stuart had a lovely wedding.

WHAT WERE YOUR EARLY LIVES LIKE?

Donna

Donna is from a family originally consisting of three sons and one daughter. One brother died in infancy, and with Donna being much younger than her two surviving brothers, her parents were very protective of her. She had a lonely childhood, with not much affection being shown to her by her parents or brothers. Her upbringing was strict, and she received much verbal abuse, mainly from her mother. As a result, Donna describes herself as having a low self-esteem, poor confidence, and a tendency to downgrade herself.

> * Her original low self-esteem has made it easier for Donna to take a submissive role in her marriage to Stuart. Over the years, however, she has gradually learned to express her desires.

Since she had few opportunities to socialize with men, when a friend of the family did show an interest in her, she quickly married to leave home. She was 34 years younger than her husband. Her mother strongly objected to the marriage. When Donna's father and mother died, her two brothers managed to acquire most of the family's assets, leaving little for Donna. In recent years, she has had contact with her brothers. They like Stuart and have given her some of her mother's jewelry and household items.

> * Donna was so confined and controlled as a young woman that the only man she could meet was a family friend who visited the home. Being married to a much older man reinforced the childlike role she assumed in her family of origin. In this role it was difficult for her to fight her more powerful older brothers for her rightful inheritance.

In high school she studied clerical skills and held secretarial positions during much of her adult working years.

Stuart

Stuart was one of eight children in a close-knit family. He had a wonderful childhood with many interesting activities. His father worked in construction, and both parents died many years ago. Apparently Stuart liked adventure, because at age 18 he left home, joining the Merchant Marines and traveling around the world. When he returned home, he earned a degree as a chemical engineer.

Stuart was employed for many years as an engineer for a petroleum company, often traveling to the company's overseas facilities. At age 60 he retired from full-time work but continued consulting in other countries until age 65.

WHAT WERE YOUR PREVIOUS RELATIONSHIPS LIKE?

Donna

When Donna met her first husband, she was 26 and he was 60. He was a calm, quiet, easy-going man, and they had a good relationship. After 25 years of marriage, he died from pneumonia. They had no children, although Donna had always wanted to be a mother. A medical misdiagnosis had resulted in a hysterectomy that prevented pregnancy.

Stuart

Stuart married at age 21, and this marriage lasted for 56 years. He had one daughter and two sons. His marriage was a good one. His wife was ill with cancer for seven years and died shortly before his relationship with Donna started.

WHAT ADJUSTMENTS HAVE YOU MADE?

It is interesting to follow the fluctuations in the balance of power in this relationship. As with most traditional marriages of older folks, Donna and Stuart's marriage is, for the most part, male controlled. Not only custom and religious convictions have supported Stuart's dominance in the marriage. His income is considerably larger than Donna's, so he holds the purse strings and has the final veto over major financial decisions. For example, Donna would like to sell Stuart's house, now a rental, putting the proceeds into a larger home. This would allow her to have more space for their things, including a separate office area for herself. She believes, as she said, "It would be easier to take care of a larger home." When I asked Stuart about this idea, he replied that Donna would not be able to care for a larger home as she got older. That seemed to settle the matter.

Donna receives Social Security benefits and earns some money by free-lancing secretarial services. As she puts it, "I can use this money for things I want that Stuart doesn't think I need."

> * It is good that Donna has a small income of her own. It gives her some independence and ability to satisfy her "wants." Money is an important determinant of power in a relationship.

One major difference that required attention was the maintenance of an acceptable temperature in their house. Stuart never seemed to feel heat or cold. It took some time for Donna to make him aware that she felt the cold and that a suitable fire should be maintained in the living room fireplace. After repeated complaints from her, he learned to accommodate her need for warmth.

Another major conflict between them was that Stuart never seemed to get hungry, getting by often on one, or at the most, two meals a day. On the other hand, Donna frequently felt hungry or even "starved," as Stuart did not suggest that it was time to eat. Gradually as she learned to make her needs known, Stuart listened, and they now have meals at regular times.

> * Donna was so downtrodden in her childhood that she initially lacked the conviction that her own desires were important. She gradually has learned to speak up.

Before their marriage Donna had a number of dogs and cats in the house and on the grounds. At one time she considered three cats as "her babies." Stuart was both allergic to the cats and uncomfortable with them. Despite this Donna told him, "I've had them longer than I've had you!" Now Donna has a single cat, and Stuart has overcome his allergy. He even likes this cat and takes care of it when Donna is away from home but is not always confident that he is doing the job properly. He admits he doesn't have "the mother instinct."

> * Here Donna was able to be assertive, at least to keep one cat; this despite Stuart's allergy. The cat, "her baby," was important enough to stand up for.

Donna and Stuart have compromised equally in many areas. At the very beginning of their marriage, Stuart made the major concession in giving up his home for Donna's. Each one had complete furnishings, and it was difficult for both of them to part with many objects that could not fit into their one home. They each gave up some loved possessions. Even now, their house feels cluttered because each of them has items with which they could not part.

> * It is really hard to part with precious possessions, many of them holding fond memories. You often see every

surface covered in the homes of older couples who married when they were young. So imagine having to combine these many items in the home of a newly coupled older couple.

Donna is disturbed when Stuart leaves a large kitchen light on, does not close the toilet seat cover, and doesn't wash dishes to her satisfaction. He has gradually changed his habits. Now Donna does the dishes more often!

* I'm glad to see that Stuart has changed habits to please Donna. Since she is particular, it is good that she does the dishes herself rather than criticize Stuart.

Stuart thinks at times that Donna spends too much money on unnecessary items. She likes to stock up on household materials since the stores at which they shop are at a distance from their house. The quantities she collects give her a secure feeling. They argue about such things at times, but she says, "I never win."

* In actuality, she does stock up on food and acquires other items she wants. She just doesn't get Stuart to agree it's the right thing to do. She wins but doesn't realize she wins. Like Donna, women throughout history have gained their power in subtle ways, often without acknowledging to themselves that they did so.

Donna is aware that, as Stuart slows down with age, she supports him in many ways, more than she would like him to know. This is beginning to somewhat change the balance of power in this marriage. For example, she has done all the driving for the past three years, as Stuart is now unable to drive as a result of his general weakness.

He finds it hard to accept that his physical strength is waning, and although Donna helps him with such chores as bringing in the wood and clearing the yard, she doesn't make a point of it.

> * Thus, Donna keeps up the appearance of the traditional role, protecting Stuart's pride as he grows more dependent. This speaks of her loving consideration for him.

WHAT ARE YOUR ON-GOING ACTIVITIES?

This couple enjoys many activities, sharing responsibilities and pleasures on a fairly equal basis. In the past, because of Stuart's extensive experiences overseas, they took tours to European and South American countries. But now with Stuart having difficulty walking, such trips are over. Donna helps in their church with secretarial services and Sunday School teaching. Stuart continues to be proud of her abilities. He helps out at the church's second-hand store.

At home they read, usually the Bible and other sacred publications, watch conservative television programs together, and enjoy playing the game of Dominos. They joke together with few inhibitions.

They have many friends from their church with whom they have weekly potluck lunches. Also, they still have a few remaining friends from each one's previous marriage. At times, they both talk about these marriages. Donna likes to show pictures of her early family and her first husband. Stuart finds no fault with this.

Donna appreciates Stuart's warmly expressed affection. He reminisces that "After 56 years with my first wife, I have learned how to handle a woman to keep her loving me. Not a day goes by now that I don't put my arms around Donna a dozen times and tell her how much I love her. I never go to bed without kissing her and wishing her a good sleep."

FINAL THOUGHTS

This marriage is what I would term complementary, in that Stuart's and Donna's personalities complement each other. Stuart is a very strong, assertive man and, despite his advanced age, is very much in charge of the household. This, and his frequently expressed affection, fulfills Donna's needs to be loved and cared for. Their strong conservative religious beliefs, and both their upbringings, support the male-dominated balance of this marriage.

With Donna's very sheltered childhood, she is able to accept the more submissive role, though not without some discomfort and some assertion of her own needs, such as keeping her cat and stocking up on food. Because she is so much younger than Stuart, whose strength is beginning to fail, she is able to care for him in physical ways, such as driving the car and bringing in wood for the fireplace. Thus, the balance of power is changing somewhat as Stuart ages and he becomes more dependent on Donna. With their loving respect for and consideration of each other, this marriage continues to be a satisfactory one for them both.

Chapter 6

(Interview: Ellen and Ralph)

IT'S NOT ALL PEACHES AND CREAM ... BUT THEY'RE SURE DOING BETTER!

They met through a personal ad. After 10 months they married and moved into his home. Now, when interviewed two and a half months after their wedding, they are recognizing the need to make adjustments. What are the problems they face? How are they attempting to overcome them? Let's look at their on-going efforts for success.

THEME
The Importance of Constructive Problem-Solving

All couples have some degree of conflict between them. Ellen and Ralph have been able to look at the ways their conflict develops, show understanding of each other's situations and feelings, and take responsibility for their own behavior. This constructive problem-solving needs to be a continuing process in all successful older-couple relationships.

INTRODUCING ELLEN AND RALPH

It looked from the exterior like a large hotel set in an exclusive suburb. Entering its elegantly furnished lobby, I was greeted by the doorman. He phoned Ellen, who a few minutes later, ushered me into a spacious apartment where, over morning tea, our interview commenced.

I was not to meet Ralph until that afternoon, when Ellen introduced me to him, prior to my interviewing him alone. Seeing them together, I was struck by what an attractive pair they were. They looked as if they had just walked off a movie set, playing a typical older American couple. Both Ellen and Ralph are tall and slim, with full heads of white hair, Ellen's elegantly coifed. She wore a stylish, full-length yellow dress, and Ralph looked most handsome in well-tailored slacks and a short-sleeved summer shirt.

Ellen is 62 years old; Ralph is 69. Both are employed full time, Ellen as a real estate agent and Ralph as an insurance adjuster, though he was between jobs when we met. They are an example of a couple, who having been together just a little more than a year, are still in the working-out phase of their relationship. They have learned from past mistakes and have the intelligence and knowledge to look objectively at the difficulties in their relationship and to take steps to improve it.

HOW DID YOU MEET?

Both Ellen and Ralph had previous marriages. They had now reached a time in their lives when each was motivated to find a new partner with whom to spend their remaining years together.

Ellen had placed a notice in the personal column of her local newspaper, stating that she was "a 61-year-old female, with a good sense of humor, interested in meeting a gentleman in his 60s who likes living in a recreational-vehicle and traveling together."

During an airplane flight, Ralph talked with a psychologist sitting next to him about his interest in meeting a woman. The psychologist suggested that he look through the personal ads in the newspaper for someone of interest to him. The phone call from Ralph was one of three that Ellen received in her phone mailbox.

After a follow-up phone conversation, Ellen agreed to meet with Ralph for coffee.

> * Meeting for coffee is standard when people meet after answering an ad. It is safe and if necessary, can be brief. It wasn't brief for Ellen and Ralph.

A few days later they went together to a movie. It was so bad they walked out and went to dinner. Things seemed to go right between them, as they talked for *four hours* over their food! Shortly thereafter, Ellen asked Ralph to drive with her to visit a friend in a nearby city. He agreed, and their relationship started to develop.

> * A real compliment. You really must like someone to introduce him or her to a friend so soon.

HOW WERE YOU ATTRACTED TO EACH OTHER?

Ellen saw Ralph as a handsome man, easy to talk to, with a calm manner and a sense of humor. Ralph was attracted to Ellen by her good looks and a manner that demonstrated intelligence, sensitivity, competence, and a caring attitude. Ellen pointed out that in many ways, she and Ralph, in both looks and interests, "are reflections of ourselves."

Beyond these physical and intellectual characteristics, they discovered similarities in their backgrounds and interests. They were both brought up on Midwest farms. They have almost an equal number of children (Ellen – three, Ralph – four) and they have similar ethical standards. Equally important was each one's desire to travel in an RV and eventually live in a large one. In fact, this might have been the "clincher" for them.

HOW DID YOUR RELATIONSHIP DEVELOP?

Ellen and Ralph, who were both working full time, depended on the telephone in order to stay in contact during the week. Sometimes their conversations lasted as long as three hours. On weekends they dated, engaging in many different activities together, and visiting each other's homes.

Two months after meeting, they became sexually involved, and four months later they agreed to live together in Ralph's larger apartment condominium, this despite the fact that Ellen had to commute 45 minutes to work each day. A striking example of their compatibility was that Ellen thought she could have chosen most of Ralph's furnishings herself. She simply added some of her own furniture, and she was ready to move in. Ralph allowed her to do whatever she wished in the apartment to help her feel at home.

Each of them understood that, considering their ages, and the fact that they "had been around the block a few times," they both knew they were starting on a serious, long-term relationship that included marriage. In Ralph's words, "we didn't want to wait!"

During our discussion, I asked this question: "What were your reasons for getting married, rather than just continuing to live together." These were their answers:

"This is a long-term commitment for both persons rather than just being a convenience. In marriage we are more committed to resolve differences so that our union lasts." (Ralph)

"He fills a spot for me that has been empty for many years. I feel life becomes much more meaningful with marriage, and there is a purpose now beyond just existence." (Ellen)

Four months after starting to live together, Ellen and Ralph were married in Hawaii.

WHAT WERE YOUR PREVIOUS RELATIONSHIPS LIKE?

Ellen

Ellen has had three previous marriages. She was first wedded at age 20. This lasted for 11 years and they had three children. Her husband became an alcoholic and physically abusive. After 10 years, Ellen remarried. This union lasted for two-and-a-half years, ending when her husband died from a sudden heart attack. While not an ideal husband, he was good with the children. His unexpected death was difficult for her.

Following this marriage, Ellen developed a relationship with a friend of her second husband, and they married after a year. Their marriage was more of a good friendship than a love match. It lasted for six months, but as Ellen said, "Without love, no matter how hard we tried, our marriage had no fulfilling aspects." It ended with a mutual divorce.

For the next 16 years, Ellen lived alone, although she had some passing relationships. It was during this period that she became financially self-supporting in various occupations, including property management, marketing, and now in real estate.

Ralph

Ralph also had three previous marriages. The first one, at age 26, was to a woman who later developed breast cancer that remained untreated until Ralph insisted that she see a doctor. The irony is that she was a registered nurse. After six years of what was proving to be a good marriage, with four children, Ralph's first wife passed away. Six months after his wife's death, he married a much younger woman. A widower with four children, he entered this marriage out of desperation. His new wife was far too young and inexperienced to be a stepmother to the children. After four difficult months, they divorced.

Ralph married for the third time five years later. During this period, he was a bus driver, and was required to be away from home much of the time. This absence affected the marriage, which ended in four years.

WHAT PROBLEMS WERE FACED AND WHAT ADJUSTMENTS WERE MADE?

When Ellen and Ralph first met, they "clicked" with each other. Many things just matched between them and provided a good start for their relationship. Their positive attitude continued as they lived together and then married. Now, within the last six months, problems have arisen.

First, Ellen, in addition to her 45-minute commute to work each way, puts in many hours of work selling real estate, including evenings and weekends. She often comes home quite exhausted. Understandably, she wants more help from Ralph.

Second, in recent months, Ralph has changed insurance adjusting jobs, and at the time of our interview, was in the middle of a three-week period between positions. In addition, he went through a traumatic operation for cancer not too long ago.

> * Job security forms an essential part of a person's self-esteem. Even with a new position in sight, the lay-off period could certainly have negatively affected Ralph. An operation for cancer is an extremely stressful life event. I

believe Ralph must have been experiencing some degree of depression. Depression affects the ability to be as fully active and involved as Ellen would have liked.

Now, let us examine some of their present conflicts and see how Ellen and Ralph are attempting to overcome them.

Views from Ellen's Perspective

"Over the past six months, I've become more responsible for what goes on in our marriage—housekeeping, chores, making purchases, cooking dinners, social activities. This was not true when we first started dating and then living together. I resent having to handle all these responsibilities alone."

* It is good that Ellen is aware of her resentment. Thus, she can express it directly to Ralph. If an individual is unaware of underlying resentment, it can be expressed indirectly in hurtful ways such as withdrawal or sarcasm.

"Ralph is between jobs. He may be depressed and insecure as to where he is going."

* Here Ellen shows understanding of Ralph's probable depression. The ability to sense and appreciate your spouse's underlying emotions is extremely important.

"I am cast in the leadership role because I'm so competent, but my husband is extremely competent himself. He's capable of doing as much as I can. I would like him to take more responsibility on his part and also initiate activities together with me."

* Instead of putting Ralph down, she gives him credit for being competent. She's clear about what she wants.

Views from Ralph's Perspective

"She has very definite feelings about how she wants to be treated."

* Ellen is clear about what she wants, and he hears her—a good sign.

"I attribute ulterior motives to what she says."

* He is aware that he is attributing. In other words, he knows that Ellen may or may not have "ulterior motives."

"Maybe we should have waited longer to be married to better understand each other."

* They could have had a longer period of living together to work out problems before marriage, as Jerry and I did. But whether living together or married, couples usually need some time to make the first adjustments. Ellen and Ralph strongly wanted the commitment of marriage.

WORKING THINGS OUT

I first interviewed Ellen and Ralph separately. The next morning, I met with them together. During the previous evening, they had obviously begun to work on the problems between them. Each one made a number of frank and sincere statements that included the following:

By Ellen

"When we get into an argument, we must decide how we're going to work things out. Part of solving an argument is to bond and create an intimacy together."

* Very true.

"Both of us understand that because we are such independent personalities, we can become brutal verbally, and that could destroy our marriage. Therefore, we have to find a way to change. One way is through some type of signal to indicate that a dangerous blowup is coming, then separating until we calm down."

* They have begun to do this, and it works!

"We certainly have similar goals, and one thing I've noticed about Ralph is that when he knows how I feel about something, he will do anything to make things better between us."

* She gives him credit for wanting to please her.

"It's hard for him to read my mind when all he sees or hears is an emotional reaction from me. I must consciously overcome that behavior."

* Here Ellen takes responsibility for her own actions. She knows she must control her emotions. She needs to state her point clearly when she is calmer. And she's right—no one can read minds.

"I love him very much, and I am very committed to do anything I can to make this a successful marriage, but I can't do it by myself. I know he's also very committed to our relationship. I need him to reassure me of that."

* We all need reassurance that we are loved and that the relationship is of prime importance. Ellen is openly asking for reassurance and giving Ralph credit for his commitment to her.

By Ralph

"I've had bad situations before and don't want them to happen again. Sometimes my baggage from previous relationships makes me suspicious. I must learn not to let previous relationships color this relationship."

* He is taking responsibility for his own reactions.

"We say things in anger to each other that can be hurtful. She internalizes things that at a later time come bubbling out. They may have no importance or real meaning. I must not take them so seriously."

* In wishing to be less hurt when Ellen explodes, he acknowledges that he has some control over his own emotions. It is more constructive to understand and change your own responses than to try to change your partner's behavior.

"Ellen is absolutely right. We must stop such brutal arguments, because at some point, they could tip us over, and neither of us wants that."

* In my work with couples, I give rules for arguing. They need to learn *not* to threaten to leave and *not* to call each other unkind names. Ellen and Ralph are learning such rules and are starting to take a "time out" if they think they are losing control. Unless these rules are followed, hurt and bitterness builds up and threatens a marriage. Ralph's statement shows an understanding of this danger.

"I am really convinced Ellen internalizes things until they get to the point at which they explode. If she could tell me at the time, when I am insulting, demeaning, irritating, or disrespectful of her, that would be a big help. I would then be able to cope with it right then."

* Here Ralph is willing to admit that he can be insulting. He also hits on another key point. Rather than let hurt and anger build up slowly, it is important to express what disturbs you as soon as possible in a non-blaming way. Ellen could say to Ralph, using an "I" statement, "I feel hurt by your tone of voice. Could you say that to me in a different way?"

"Both of us love each other enough to do what's necessary to get past some of these blocks and make this relationship work."

* This mirrors Ellen's last statement about commitment. Both of them want to make the marriage work and to have a good understanding of the problems in their interactions.

FINAL OBSERVATIONS

Ellen and Ralph are an excellent example of the early adjustment stage, common in most new relationships. When interviewed, they had not known each other for as long a time as had many of the other couples described in this book. They still needed time to understand and accommodate each other's needs and personalities. Of course, it is a bit arbitrary to ascribe the working out of problems to an early adjustment stage only. Life is continually changing, especially as we age. (**Naomi** and **David's** situation is a good example of this.)

I contacted Ellen and Ralph sometime after our interview and learned that they were still actively involved in constructive problem-solving. And very recently, a postcard from them, while traveling and permanently living in their motor home, reads, "We're enjoying our retirement and continuing to make adjustments."

The process of constructive problem-solving never stops. It includes clear communication, careful listening to your partner, and striving to understand his or her point of view. Important also are stating your own desires in a clear non-blaming way, and taking responsibility for your own motivations, feelings, and behaviors. All of this, Ellen and Ralph continue to do. With their love for each other and their determination to make their marriage work, they are well on their way to a good life together.

Chapter 7

(Interview: Gayle and Jim)

SHE'S 10 YEARS OLDER ... IT'S WORKING FINE

Can age make a difference? Gayle and Jim say it affects more people around them than it affects them. Once, when they were with friends, a man asked Jim, "She's a lot older that you, isn't she?" Jim replied, "If *I* were older than *she*, you'd never ask that question."

THEME
Thank the Goddess ... They Found Each Other

Both Gayle and Jim, spiritual in an unconventional sense, appealed to their guiding spirits for a mate and received what they asked for. Gayle, who told her Goddess specifically what she wanted in a man, was able to recognize Jim when he walked in the door.

Knowing what you really want in a partner, and not being willing to settle for less, can sometimes, in a magical way, bring you what you desire.

Gayle and Jim met me at a county road to guide me to their house five miles away. It was a winding, hilly, bumpy drive over dirt roads through rocky California foothills, just beginning to turn green from the winter rains. About the time I began wondering, "How far must it be?" there appeared a large, gracious redwood house, lined with trees, set by a river, and with smoke coming from the chimney.

The house is open and spacious, with the living room having a high ceiling, hardwood floors, and a large rock-faced fireplace. A large outside deck overlooks the river and rocky, oak-covered hills. A few metal sculptured pieces by Gayle are displayed inside and outside the house.

INTRODUCING GAYLE AND JIM

Gayle, a 59-year-old widow, is a sculptor and the owner of a small art gallery. She is of medium height, size 14 (as she described herself), with silver hair and an open, friendly, talkative manner. She was dressed in jeans and a colorful shirt over which she wore an attractive beaded necklace.

Jim, 10 years younger, and divorced, is a writer, free-lance editor, and skilled in computers. He also is of medium height, somewhat stout, with brown hair and eyes and a ruddy, smiling face. He was dressed casually in colorful pants and a T-shirt.

Lively and affectionate, Gayle frequently touched Jim's arm or leg and kissed him on the cheek. He then smiled at her lovingly.

The 95 acres on which the house sits is owned by Gayle. In addition to the house, Gayle has a studio in which she creates metal and stone sculptures. Gayle and Jim live here together, planning to get married in six months. As our conversation started, I could hear soft, gentle classical music coming from speakers mounted high on the walls.

HOW DID YOU MEET?

One morning, five years ago, Gayle was in her art gallery and Jim came in. She spent about two hours telling him about the displays and the gallery operation. When lunchtime came, he agreed to pick up lunch for them, and they continued talking. Finally he purchased some art as gifts and made a phone call to friends in the community whom Gayle also knew. Gayle thought, "I think this guy is flirting with me. He looks very, very cute and certainly is younger than me."

The friends he called came to the gallery and, much to Gayle's surprise, Jim warmly hugged the lady. According to Gayle, "He did it very nicely. I'd better not let him out of my sight!"

At the same time, Jim thought to himself, "I want to know her better than just as a proprietor of a gallery."

> * Here Gayle and Jim, by spending such a long time conversing, gained a good idea of the other's intellect, interests, and values. And it was their mutual attraction that led them to prolong their visit and learn so much about each other.

Gayle invited the friends to dinner a month later and asked Jim to come also. She prepared a sumptuous dinner. Jim brought wine, and Gayle observed how well he interacted with their mutual friends. As Gayle knew that Jim was skilled with computers, she asked him for help with one she had recently acquired. He happily agreed to go to her house to help her.

WHAT ATTRACTED YOU TO EACH OTHER?

As Gayle started to live alone after her husband's death, she became lonely, wanting to share her life with someone. A devotee to the Goddess religion, at 2:00 one morning, with a full moon in sight, she went up on a special hill near the house to ask her Goddess for help.

She asked for someone to love, one who would love her, but just not anyone. Her Goddess then asked what she was looking for and Gayle replied, "A man who is not a drinker or smoker, intelligent, educated, open-minded. Since I've accomplished a lot in my life, I don't want someone threatened by my successes, but delighted with what I've accomplished. He should like animals and be kind to dogs and cats. He should be self-sufficient and not want me to care for him at this stage of life. While comfortable with me, he should have his own interests in life, be nurturing, compassionate, and with no hang-ups about sex. Finally, he should be concerned about the community in which we live."

Gayle found the following qualities in Jim: "He has a wonderful, open, smiling face with lively eyes—a warm person. He doesn't seem to be a 'game player.' He doesn't try to impress me with his work or with his previous relationships with women. He seems self-sufficient and has his own interests in life. He is a compassionate person, very trusting, open, and honest."

Jim described features that he found attractive in Gayle: "Her liveliness and enthusiasm. The way she approaches life. She's very positive. I feel no age difference in her presence."

These were qualities that Gayle and Jim both knew they wanted in a partner and that Gayle so specifically enumerated to her Goddess.

* You might want to write down the traits that are important to you, as suggested in Section Three, *How Do You Find a Partner?* Or you might know these traits on some level and thus, be able to recognize them in another person. To protect yourself from becoming involved with the wrong person, it is just as important to recognize such behaviors that are opposite of those that Gayle observed in Jim, such as "game playing," boasting, and being overly dependent on others.

HOW DID YOUR RELATIONSHIP DEVELOP?

After the first dinner party, Jim came from the city to Gayle's house to give her some help with her computer. As Gayle recounted, "When he entered my house, my dog, who never shows an interest in any man, came right over to Jim. When he kneeled down to pet her, she actually licked his face. I've never seen that before! Then, to top it off, my cat, who is very independent, came to his chair, allowing him to pick her up. This fellow really has something special!"

> * Even the animals were quick to see that there was something special about Jim. This would fit with Gayle's belief that animals have a special intelligence and ability to judge the good and bad in humans.

"We had a five-hour visit that evening," Gayle continued. "When he left, he gave me a hug. It felt very good."

Gayle didn't hear from Jim for a month. Then she received an attractive hand-designed thank-you card. He included his telephone number, fax number, pager number, and e-mail address. This list certainly seemed very inviting to Gayle! A few days later, she phoned to tell him she was going to the city and that she'd like to stop by his apartment to see his computer equipment. She jokingly said she would take some fast food, but instead she cooked a gourmet dinner, and to be prepared, she took her toothbrush and a package of condoms with her.

That evening she found a very neat apartment (although somewhat later she saw that his bedroom, in which the computer equipment was located, was very messy) and a table set attractively with wine glasses in place. Jim had a fire blazing in the fireplace, and Mozart quietly filled the room. Two friendly cats greeted her. Gayle was positively impressed.

After they ate, Jim brought out a deck of Tarot cards. Both Jim and Gayle believe that Tarot cards can predict the future. Jim's thought was, "Let's see what God set in my lap."

Much to their surprise (and pleasure!) the cards that each selected and played showed fortunes in each other's favor!

"Do you know what this means?" asked Gayle.

"I think so," was the reply.

"Then why don't you invite me to spend the night?"

"Sounds good to me."

At this point, Jim's thought was, "Is this what I've prayed for—someone special for me?"

> * Though he might not have been as specific in his prayer as Gayle was to her Goddess, Jim has the strong belief that his entreaty to a higher power helped bring Gayle to him. I believe that many happy couples have the conviction that God helped them find each other. **Laura** has faith that a divine being helped form her union with **Ed**.

They had a very good night together. "The most wonderful ever. He's very knowledgeable about sex," confided Gayle.

The next night Jim phoned Gayle to thank her for visiting. Since she had forgotten to look at his computer the previous evening (did she really forget?), she agreed to return that night ... and again the next night. Then after the weekend that they spent at her house, she suggested, "How about a permanent relationship?" Jim agreed.

A few weeks later Gayle told Jim that she had a one-month trip to Mexico coming up. Her son was married to a Mexican woman, and she had planned to visit them. Jim agreed to stay in her house to take care of the animals and watch over things while she was gone. At that time, Jim had a regular job as an editor for a magazine, requiring an hour-and-a-half commute to work for him each day. But to him, it all seemed worth the effort. A few days after Gayle left, this became questionable when a big storm flooded the road and caused some landslides that made travel treacherous. Yet, he stayed on and persisted in caring for Gayle's home and getting to work.

> * Though Gayle, who has the more assertive personality, did much to initiate the relationship, Jim certainly was deeply interested. Why else would he commute an hour-and-a-half daily and brave floods and landslides to care for Gayle's property?

When Gayle returned from her trip, they both realized that neither one enjoyed being apart. Therefore, Jim agreed to make a permanent move into Gayle's house. As he settled in, Jim thought he'd like to get married right away. To him marriage meant, "a formal legal commitment. With a ten-year age difference, marriage gives us a firm ground of love and commitment together."

Gayle said, "I could live like this the rest of my life, but I know marriage is important since other people see it as a permanent, legitimate relationship."

When they discussed wedding plans, Gayle explained that she would be 60 years old in a few months and until that age it would not be practical for her to be married. The reason to wait was in order to qualify for Social Security benefits from her deceased husband's account. The law states that if she were to remarry before age 60, she would lose all payments, but after 60 she could start to receive payments when she reached 62. With this consideration, they planned the wedding to take place after her sixtieth birthday.

WHAT WERE YOUR EARLY YEARS LIKE?

Gayle

Gayle was the youngest of five children in a poor, struggling family that was native to the area in which she now lives. Her father was a farmer, and on the side, a musician. He was an alcoholic and physically abused her mother. Gayle, as a child, was sexually molested by an uncle. Gayle's parents quarreled constantly, and she left home at age 10 to live with an aunt and to stay with other families until she could become independent. In many of the homes where she lived, the men attempted to sexually molest her, but she fought them off.

I asked Gayle how she managed to survive such a childhood. "I had an aunt who said I was a 'changeling.' This meant I was really a gypsy child brought into the family. From a very early age, I thought I was an ancient spirit in a child's body so that I could watch what was happening in my family and not be a part of it. In the second grade I began to read Greek myths, and they became part of my fantasy life. Often during the summer, I would retreat to a special private spot under a bridge by a creek near our home. There I could look up at the creek, see the butterflies and flowers, and hear the bubbling pool beneath. Then I could commune with my protectors, the Good Fairy and the Greek Goddess, *Artemis*. Another of my protectors was from the comic strip, *Wonder Woman.* Wonder Woman's mother was the Goddess *Minerva* who lived on Mt. Olympus. With these protectors, I was not a part of the fighting and chaos in my home. Sometimes I would draw pictures of these powerful women or mold little clay statues of them to keep near my bed."

* Gayle is a perfect example of the "transcendent child" as presented by Rubin in her book of the same name.

This book describes individuals who had horrendous childhoods and not only survived them, but as does Gayle, excelled as adults.

Rubin uses the term "disidentification," which literally means "not identifying with." The adults she describes could look clearly at their families' crazy behaviors and not blame themselves or feel unworthy. To quote Rubin, "Their distance and disidentification enables them to construct their own narrative—a story that separated them from the pathology around them; a story that in every case underscored the boundary between them and me" (Lillian B. Rubin, *The Transcendent Child* (1996), HarperCollins Publishers, page 226).

As a child, Gayle, through her fantasies, did exactly this, creating a narrative that separated her from her family and helped her grow into a happy and successful adult. People who have had terrible childhoods are often strongly spiritual, as is Gayle. Their beliefs help them to survive as children and continue to give strength in their adult lives.

Jim

Jim's family was not an affectionate one. His father had an alcohol problem but was able to manage a restaurant and be both a painter and a sculptor. Jim's mother was a secretary for many years. He grew up with one sister.

From an early age, Jim wrote poetry and short stories. His parents were proud of these accomplishments, and he dreamed of being a writer when he grew up. He later graduated from college with a major in English and creative writing. After some difficult years with frequent unemployment, he found work as an editor for a well-known magazine.

WHAT WERE YOUR PREVIOUS RELATIONSHIPS LIKE?

Gayle

At age 14, while a high school sophomore, Gayle met her husband-to-be, who was 10 years older. They were married two years later, when she was 16. Their marriage lasted 38 years.

After marrying and finishing high school, Gayle completed a two-year course at an art institute, majoring in sculpture. She then stayed home for 10 years, raising two daughters, and sculpting in a studio her husband had built for her. When the children were older, she became an assistant manager of a department store. Eventually, she completed a master's degree in business administration. This advanced education led to employment as an administrator in a branch of a large corporation and eventually to opening her own art gallery, thus combining her business expertise with her love of art. She soon became involved in many community activities and remains so to this day. She joined the Chamber of Commerce, serving as president for several years. She has helped sponsor the girls' soccer league, and has volunteered to teach sculpture in the local community center.

> * Gayle's energy and enthusiasm are almost overwhelming to me. Learning of her activities today, I can visualize her as a young teenager, working as a maid and baby-sitter in one of her many abusive foster homes, and fighting off the husband's sexual advances. This took strength and self-possession, qualities she still has.

Gayle's husband started as a technician with an automotive company. He rose to an administrative position, becoming financially well off. They had a good, mutually supportive marriage for 28 years.

According to Gayle, her husband always gave her what she wanted materially. For the last 10 years of their marriage, he developed a serious drinking problem. Although he was not abusive while drinking, this matter seriously affected their marriage, including making him sexually impotent. During this time, Gayle tried to help him but to no avail.

> * Impotence is a frequent result of heavy drinking. Trying to "help" an alcoholic never works. The person must recognize his problem and seek treatment himself. I refer spouses or other family members of serious drinkers to Alanon. There they learn to stop "enabling" behaviors, such as when the alcoholic has a hangover, calling the workplace to say that the spouse is too sick to work. Alanon also teaches participants how to avoid having their lives consumed by the drinking problem and how to take care of themselves within the relationship.

Early in their marriage, Gayle had been deeded the land from her mother that she and Jim now live on. She and her husband decided to build a house on the property. Gayle took charge of the project, planning an energy-efficient house, and the construction started. They never lived together in their new house, as suddenly, before it was completed, her husband had a fatal heart attack. This was quite a shock to Gayle and as we spoke, tears came to her eyes. (Her husband's ashes are in a jar on a shelf in the living room.)

> * Twenty-eight years of a stable, caring relationship (even with her husband's drinking problem) started when Gayle was only 16. He encouraged her in her many activities and accomplishments, and this was certainly a great support to Gayle. It is a credit to her good sense as a young

woman that she was able to select such a man, and over the years sustain a stable marriage, raising two children. I remark on this because of Gayle's terrible childhood. People can overcome the wounds of childhood and lead productive, happy lives.

Gayle concluded this discussion by saying, "Then I dated some nice men, and if I had been responsive, I could have married any one of them. But I was not going to settle for less than I really wanted. Also, I really missed having a good sexual relationship." She told me she was not sexually involved with any of these men. A year and a half after her husband died, Gayle met Jim. She strongly believes that her husband's spirit guided Jim to her.

* After her husband's death, although she had many opportunities, Gayle was not willing to settle for less that she desired in a partner. Knowing specifically what she wanted in a mate helped her to be ready for Jim. Her continued love for her husband, and her belief that he wished her happiness, gave her the confidence that he, along with her Goddess, brought Jim to her.

Jim

Jim's sister, while in college, had a roommate whom he met when he was 20 years old. He married her two years later, and the marriage lasted 13 years. They had one child, a son. Throughout the marriage, Jim and his wife had difficulties supporting each other emotionally. His wife wanted him to be like her father who had an entirely different way of life. She resented being the sole breadwinner during Jim's periods of unemployment. Jim became depressed and "felt isolated as in a cave."

As time went on, Jim's and his wife's differences increased, and their arguments became more frequent and more bitter. Jim said, "I didn't understand a lot of the things she needed. I was being an ass. If I had the opportunity to do it over again, I'd not make the same mistakes again."

> * That Jim could take responsibility for the breakup of his marriage, rather than blame his wife, impressed Gayle very favorably. It "takes two to tango," and in any failed relationship, it is important to look at your own behavior as well as that of your ex-spouse. In that way, you can learn and grow so the next relationship will not have the same pitfalls.

Finally his wife filed for divorce. After the divorce, Jim's depression changed to a negative and cynical attitude toward life, which now that he is with Gayle, has gradually been replaced with positive emotions.

In the interim, before meeting Gayle, Jim had brief affairs with a number of women. Nothing serious developed. Before his relationship with Gayle became sexual, he had an AIDS test.

> * This is important for older individuals before becoming sexually involved. Infection with AIDS is alarmingly high in the over-50 population. This may be because so many unattached older adults are sexually active.

WHAT PROBLEMS WERE FACED AND WHAT ADJUSTMENTS WERE MADE?

When I asked Gayle and Jim about problems encountered in their relationship, their immediate comments were: "I don't believe we've made many changes. On further thought, I suppose we have made some minor adjustments. It's difficult to identify any problems we've had except for little ones like Jim dumping things around the house and not picking them up. I like neatness. We don't have any arguments, but we do have discussions over differences, once in a while."

> * As with Gayle and Jim, quite a few couples I interviewed, at first could recall few, if any, problems and adjustments. As the interviews progressed, they gradually remembered or recognized difficulties they had experienced and willingly talked about them.

When I raised the question, "How does your age difference affect things between you?" I received the following responses:

Gayle explained, "I was nervous at first. I was concerned about my appearance and what his friends would think. When I prepared for a party at his office, I actually dyed my hair, used new makeup, and wore bright clothes—all to look younger. I also remember one time when we visited a museum and I noticed a woman with a young boy looking at us. I listened carefully and heard her say, 'That must be her son with her.' The young boy replied, 'No mom, that's her boyfriend.'"

> * What a perceptive child!

Then Jim added, "I never feel the age difference when I'm with Gayle. We have realized that it actually is more important to people around us than to us. Some people question why we're together. Gayle is wealthier than I am; therefore, I must have married her for her money. Not true."

"I remember one time," Jim continued, "when we were with some friends, and a man asked me, 'She's a lot older than you, isn't she?' I replied, 'If *I* were older than *she,* you'd never ask that question.' It's a question that relates to our culture and we should realize it need not be asked or even thought about."

As our talk progressed, Gayle and Jim described ways they relate to each other that makes their relationship so successful.

Gayle commented, "We're very open and honest with each other."

"Yes," replied Jim, "I've told her that if I'm doing something that really offends her to please tell me. I may or may not be able to change. Therefore, we need to talk the matter over. I screwed up my first marriage and don't want to make such a mistake again. At least she'll give me the chance."

When Jim moved into Gayle's house, she expected him to help out with many of the physical tasks necessary around the house and the grounds. These included repairing fences, cutting wood for the fireplace, trimming weeds, and other chores needed to maintain a large acreage in the country. Then she also wanted some computer work quickly completed for an organization. At first, Jim was confused. He could handle the computer work, but being a "flatlander" (hill people such as Gayle, call valley folks flatlanders), he found other tasks to be difficult. Which should be done first?

When Jim pointed out the conflict in her expectations, Gayle realized that she had to ask herself, "What's really important right now?" She decided, "We can get someone to do the outside work so Jim can spend time on what he does best, work on the computer."

Now Jim cuts firewood, trims weeds, and handles some other physical chores that he enjoys but spends most of his time on computer projects.

A major problem and consequent adjustment relates to a serious situation that Gayle described in detail. She had acquired the habit of drinking as a youth and returned to it after her husband died. Although she became a heavy drinker, she was able to continue with her many activities, and she did not acknowledge that she had a problem.

> * This is not surprising since her father, grandparents, uncle, and most of her siblings had been alcoholics. Much research supports the theory that susceptibility to alcoholism is genetic and runs in families.

One evening she and Jim, whom she encouraged to drink with her, were both quite drunk. They needed to go somewhere in the car, and she decided to drive. The result was that she ran into a tree, totaling Jim's car and causing him to suffer five broken ribs. She was arrested and faced serious legal charges. This became the "moment of awakening" for Gayle. She stopped drinking, started counseling, and attended Alcoholic Anonymous. As Gayle said, "That was the time when we started to feel more trust and honesty between us. The experience helped us to see things more accurately and clearly."

Because of her good reputation, continuing extensive community services, and her attendance at Alcoholics Anonymous, Gayle was put on probation. From then on, with additional support from Jim, she did not drink.

> * A major adjustment, right?

Gayle quotes an AA saying, "God grant me the serenity to accept the people I cannot change, the courage to change the ones I can and the wisdom to know it's ME."

* Like Gayle, it often takes an involvement with the law, or another life crisis such as loss of a job or marriage, for an individual to face his or her drinking problem. A drinker frequently associates only with other drinkers and feels quite alone when sober. Alcoholics Anonymous helps break through denial, offering the support of others who have fought the same battle, and providing a new social milieu.

Jim listened attentively as Gayle described her victory over alcoholism. After awhile he took her hand in his and said, "Before I met Gayle I had a sarcastic outlook on life. I made fun of everything. That attitude has changed as a result of living with her. I have a new way of looking at life. She brings out a more nurturing feeling in me."

At this point, he took her in his arms, and said, "I'm so grateful to you. I feel like I have a chance to be a human being again." Remaining in Jim's arms, Gayle kissed his cheek. "You let me know what makes you happy, and it's often me—just being me. That brings me much joy."

WHAT ARE YOUR ONGOING ACTIVITIES?

Gayle continues almost at "full steam" with her gallery, her sculpting, and her many volunteer activities. Jim has tried to slow her down, with little success. Everything she does gives her satisfaction, pleasure, and recognition, all of which are important to her. Jim admits that he enjoys watching Gayle accomplish things while helping other people. He also participates in some volunteer work with her.

Jim left his editing job soon after moving in with Gayle. His freelance editing work has increased, and he is deeply involved in writing a novel. He and Gayle also collaborate on projects. They both brainstorm a problem, consider and select development ideas, and then Jim completes the written work on the computer.

Though occupied with their many activities, Gayle and Jim try to control their time together. Sometimes they take a day off to relax, hang around the house, stay in bed, or go for walks. A lot can be accomplished at home because they do not watch television. Watching films on video and listening to music are good entertainment substitutes.

FINAL THOUGHTS

And so, in their rich and satisfying life together, Gayle and Jim have received what each has prayed for and what Gayle asked for in such detail from her Goddess. They knew what they wanted, and they found it. They have defied the cultural expectation that the man should be older than the woman. May they be an example to many—*vive la différence*!

Chapter 8

(Interview: Laura and Ed)

BUILDING A NEW LIFE WITH AN OLD FRIEND

"With our first mates, we lived nearby, played golf, and socialized together. Then my husband and Ed's wife each passed away within a year. A plan, like a miracle from above, brought the two of us together, leading to our joyful union. We are very fortunate."

THEME
From a Long Friendship to Marriage and Advancing Age

Friendship first, before romance, is one way to build a strong foundation. It enables a couple to learn about each other from a distance, without the expectations of a committed relationship.

Socializing as two couples, Laura and Ed were able to observe each other's interactions with their respective spouses. Then, as their friendship developed after their mates' deaths, they supported each other, sharing thoughts and feelings. The qualities they recognized in each other during this time of grieving stood them in good stead when, after many years of their own marriage, they began to deal with the difficulties of advancing age.

INTRODUCING LAURA AND ED

I walked into the elegant lobby of a large retirement facility; rode the elevator up to their floor, and walked down a long hall to the door of Laura and Ed's apartment. Both Laura and Ed greeted me, and we sat at their kitchen table to talk. The apartment is small, sunny, and pleasant. Ed's oil paintings decorate the walls.

"We don't have too much room here," said Laura, "but there is so much to do in this community that we are out a lot of the time. And also, most of our meals are provided, so we don't need a big kitchen and dining room."

Laura and Ed have been married for 19 years. Laura, age 80, is of average height, with coiffured white hair and smiling hazel eyes. At 90 years of age, Ed is a tall, heavy-set man with a head full of gray hair. Because of an irritated throat, he sounded gruff, but I was pleased to find him quite friendly, contributing much information during our interview.

Ed is a retired bank manager. Before her first marriage, Laura was a beautician, and then for many years she was a housewife and mother.

HOW DID YOU MEET AND HOW DID YOUR RELATIONSHIP DEVELOP?

When Laura and her husband moved to a retirement community many years ago, they became acquainted with Ed and his wife, who also lived there. This was first through their mutual participation in local sports, which later expanded to include social activities together. Both couples became good friends. Then, after several years, Laura's husband died suddenly of a heart attack. Ed's wife passed away from cancer nine months later.

Faced with similar sorrows, Laura and Ed helped and supported each other. At first they were just friends, with no emotional attraction. They saw each other frequently, grieved together, and comforted one another. As their lives settled down, together they went to church, played golf, shared community activities, ate dinners, and attended dances.

When Laura went by herself on an overseas cruise, Ed said, "I missed her." Laura nodded her head, saying, "I had a feeling for Ed that was more than casual. Being apart told me something. I suppose the expression, 'absence makes the heart grow fonder,' was very appropriate in this situation."

When Laura returned from the cruise, they became closer, holding hands and hugging. The need for each other continued to strengthen. "We were not getting any younger," exclaimed Laura, "so we agreed that marriage was the thing to do."

Thus, a year after Ed's loss, they were wed. Laura's daughter, who recalled the beautiful wedding her mother had arranged for her, told Laura, "Now it's my turn to do this for you!"

After his wife's death, Ed thought it was depressing to continue living in his house with so many memories. He sold the house, disposed of most of his possessions, and taking only his desk and leather lounge chair, moved into Laura's nearby larger house in the retirement community. Laura said, "Staying in my own home was important to me since women like to have their own things."

HOW WERE YOU ATTRACTED TO EACH OTHER?

Laura recognized Ed as a stable, wonderful person. She knew how faithful and dependable he was to his first wife. Her husband had been reserved and not very affectionate. Ed was a positive change for her. Therefore, she "just liked him."

Ed indicated that Laura was beautiful to look at, always happy and smiling. He thought she was very caring, someone with whom he wanted to spend the rest of his life. Now that he lives with her, he says, "She looks like an angel when she's asleep."

> * Ed, like most of the men interviewed, mentioned his partner's looks as the feature that first attracted him. Women are more variable in their initial responses. As with **Joanne**, they often recognize such characteristics as stability and trustworthiness.
>
> Ed soon noticed more than physical appearance. He also saw Laura as a caring person. She comforted him when he grieved for his wife, and now she takes care of him as his health fails.

WHAT WERE YOUR PREVIOUS RELATIONSHIPS LIKE?

Ed

Ed knew his first wife in high school. They built a close, devoted relationship during their courtship and 45 years of marriage. They had two sons. His wife was very athletic and participated in many activities with Ed. He showed me some early photos taken with her, admitting that he "still thinks about her now and then."

At age 62, Ed retired and, with his wife, moved to the retirement community where they met Laura and her husband. Two years before their move, his wife developed cancer, and she died after 10 years of illness. Ed was then 70 years old. It was a good marriage, and his wife's long illness and death were painful for Ed.

Laura

Laura was married to her first husband more than 39 years. They had a son and a daughter. Her husband was a businessman, giving her everything she wanted materially, but under the surface there were many differences and mistrusts. For her, sexual relations were not satisfactory, and she felt insecure because she was aware that he "played around" with other women. Looking back, she believes she may have been too dependent on her husband and too afraid to leave him, because as she expressed, "I could not make it on my own financially." In comparison, she now feels accepted and loved by Ed.

> ✻ I had the impression that Laura felt somewhat ashamed of not having left her husband, despite his having had several affairs during their marriage. I pointed out that this was a long time ago and things were different then. She agreed.

"In those days," she said, "women were not independent, nor did they talk about difficulties with their husbands. You were committed to the marriage, no matter what. You can't judge our behaviors then by today's standards."

Laura's husband retired at age 55, and they moved to the retirement community where they became acquainted with Ed and his wife. Her husband passed away suddenly from a heart attack when Laura was 60 years old.

WHAT ARE YOUR PRESENT LIVES LIKE?

Laura and Ed left the retirement community where they first met, for one where meals, housekeeping, and transportation are provided. This in itself an indication of their increased need to be taken care of. Despite the narrowing of their worlds as they age, Laura and Ed lead happy and active lives. Primary is their continued joy in being together, and in their small apartment they are very much together. Important also is their ability to part with earlier activities, such as golf, and still find pleasure in other less-demanding pursuits. They continue to enjoy visiting with their children and grandchildren.

Both Laura and Ed have health problems. Laura suffers from arthritis in her hands and one knee, and she has an irregular heart rhythm. Until a few years ago, she was an avid weaver, but her hands have lost their flexibility. She has hearing aids in each ear that "work fine." She treats her hearing problem with humor. "The hearing aid really helps a lot. When Ed is watching something I don't want to see on TV, I just turn off my trusty aid and continue reading."

> * What a good idea! I can't read or concentrate on anything when Jerry has the television or radio on. But fortunately (or maybe unfortunately), I don't have a hearing problem.

Ed's problems are much more limiting. He has had severe difficulty with his heart. He has had two bypass operations and two blockages removed from his arteries. He takes medication to control angina, and thus has curtailed many of his more strenuous activities. This was a gradual slowing down for a man who once was very athletic.

Because of Ed's problems with his circulatory system, he and Laura have become much more careful with their diet, consuming small amounts of red meat, more fat-free and low-cholesterol foods with little salt, and sugar-free desserts.

> * This dietary practice is slowly becoming more common among older persons as they become aware of habits for good nutrition. It has been proven that by eating more

fruits, vegetables, and grains, while reducing fats, sugars, and red meat, health can be improved.

With eating discipline, many seniors are controlling or even overcoming high blood pressure, heart conditions, potential stroke, and obesity. Those who started these practices earlier in life can see health benefits now, and I believe Ed would be having fewer problems now if he had followed this way of eating at a younger age. (See Chapter 25 for more details on nutrition and healthy living.)

Fortunately for Ed, Laura is an experienced caretaker. She began as a child by caring for her mother, who had a heart problem, and although she has had no formal training, she has nursed friends back to health over the years. She believes "Someone" is watching over her to aid her in the ability to heal. She helped herself when she suddenly suffered a serious miscarriage during her first marriage. At that time, she prayed for God's help and then felt a "presence" guiding her to health.

* Maybe this was the same ethereal support she felt when the relationship with Ed came about so naturally!

When talking about this supernatural feeling and her desire to support others, she expressed that she was, "not afraid of anything in order to assist people—I just do what I have to do." Ed agrees that Laura exhibits special powers.

* Here Laura, perhaps because of her early role of caring for her mother, now feels no resentment in caring for her husband. This is different from **Naomi**, who openly expresses resentment without guilt. We need not judge either attitude if it is comfortable for the person concerned.

Until the past few years, Laura and Ed took frequent trips to Hawaii, Europe, and elsewhere. Now traveling is too exhausting. They used to visit Laura's daughter's cabin in the mountains, but they now find the altitude difficult for their hearts. For the past six years, Laura has accepted the responsibility for all driving, as Ed suffers from macular degeneration, which has affected his eyesight.

Activities in their present retirement community have replaced much of what they have had to give up. They take trips by bus to many interesting local sites such as museums and parks. The residence's bus transports them to stores, the theater, and restaurants. They enjoy social events with the many new friends they have made in their community. Laura volunteers as a tutor in a nearby school, and a few times a week both Laura and Ed play bingo.

For many years, Ed was able to enjoy the community garden plot, growing flowers and vegetables. He visited his plot of ground several times a day during the season but now recognizes his physical limits for this activity. "I really hated giving up my garden," he said, "but life goes on."

Ed was an accomplished artist, and many of his paintings adorn their apartment walls. Now, because of macular degeneration, he no longer can paint. Giving up so much that he enjoys, first golf, then his artwork, and even his beloved gardening, has caused Ed to suffer from occasional depression. He does not allow himself to sink into lethargy. He continues to be active at home, making the bed, taking out the garbage, and helping Laura with lunches and laundry. As his ability to engage in former activities fades, he still keeps his mind active. Now he enjoys crossword puzzles, using a magnifying glass to aid his failing eyesight.

* Depression is common with increasing age, and this is understandable, given the many losses of bodily functions and previous pleasures that people experience. Continuing

to be useful at home, as does Ed, bolsters flagging self-esteem and lessens depression. We all face losses as we age, and it is important to keep our bodies as active as health permits and our minds alert.

For the mind, Ed chooses crossword puzzles, even though he must use a magnifying lens. Others might prefer playing bridge or Scrabble, taking courses at a local college, or using a computer. But as much as keeping an active mind or body, it is also important to experience positive emotions. Laura and Ed have the companionship, love, and respect for each other that help keep depression at bay and life, with advancing years, worthwhile.

FINAL THOUGHTS

A quality of friendship exists in any good relationship, whether the couple has been friends first and sweethearts later or sweethearts from the start. Many happy individuals refer to their mates as their best friends. Not all of our couples had a period of platonic friendship before they became committed. Many became romantically and sexually involved quite quickly and still have successful relationships.

It is important to fully explore issues between you and your prospective partner and then to become truly comfortable and at ease with that person. Would this person you are so attracted to at age 60 be there to care for you at age 80, as Laura cares for Ed? Would he or she be able to face the declining years with courage and dignity, as does Ed? If the answers to these questions are "yes," you and your partner will hopefully live out your years together with grace, kindness, and love.

Chapter 9

(Interview: Edna and Seymour)

WHEN MARRIED, WE'LL NEVER BE BORED!

As Edna and I talked, she told me, "I felt drawn to Seymour when we first met. Our relationship grew over the next eight months. Then Seymour decided to visit his niece in Chicago. When he returned, he told me he had met someone there and had asked her to marry him! By now, I loved him and was devastated. Even so, I still cared enough for him that I wanted him to have what he wanted. Even though he married, I had a strong premonition that he would return to me in time." And he did.

THEME
Patience and Accepting the Unexpected

Edna showed great patience and flexibility in accepting Seymour's unexpected marriage. This is not an invitation to accept a bad relationship and put life on hold, waiting for it to improve. Edna had an inner certainty based, not merely on the astrological signs she believed in, but on the reality of experiencing a good partnership with Seymour. She had the wisdom to know that men often act rashly after a wife's death and that Seymour's hasty marriage might not last. She had the patience and acceptance to be there for Seymour when he returned to her.

INTRODUCING EDNA AND SEYMOUR

Edna is 73 years of age, and Seymour is 75. He is a retired attorney, and she is a retired social worker. From the time of our first interview, they had known each other 16 years, meeting when he was 59 and she was 57. They have been married 10 years, living together 5 years before they wed. They now live in a moderate-sized, comfortably furnished condominium in a large retirement community. Edna's landscape photographs adorn the walls, and in the living room is a display of Indian arrowheads from Seymour's collection.

When I went to their home for the interview, Edna greeted me with her morning coffee in hand at 11:00. She is a late riser. She wore an iridescent violet jump suit and was limping from a pinched nerve in her leg, incurred while pushing her wheelbarrow during gardening. She has short, auburn hair, a slender build, and was friendly and direct. She believed that this interview would be "pay back" for the time when people had contributed to her requests when she was preparing her own graduate degree thesis in social welfare.

Seymour arrived about two hours later, having come directly from a doctor's appointment, dressed casually in shorts and a T-shirt. An attractive man, he has a warm, direct manner, and a magnetic quality about him. Despite his obvious intelligence, Seymour has developed a memory problem with age. Edna had to remind him of their appointment with me, and she keeps track of their busy schedules.

HOW DID YOU MEET?

Edna had been divorced four years when she met Seymour. With a lady friend, she had attended a number of dances for older singles, and she did not find any men of interest to her. She had heard of a club known as Parents Without Partners and thought that through it she might make some contacts for her youngest son. Contemplating joining, she attended a club dance.

At the gathering, Edna met Seymour beside the refreshment table. After a brief introductory conversation, she thought this man was interesting enough to ask him to dance. After a few steps, they danced closer together, and their attraction to each other started, leading to a satisfying sexual experience in her home that first night. By the way, Edna never mentioned if she found any friends for her son through this club!

HOW WERE YOU ATTRACTED TO EACH OTHER?

Seymour wanted a partner close to his own age. To him, Edna exhibited a good personality, was outgoing, and pleasant to be with.

> * It is refreshing to meet a man who explicitly states that he wants a woman close to his age. Many men seem to be looking for, or are involved with, much younger women.

Edna perceived Seymour as outgoing, a good dancer, and a very caring person. More than noticing these traits, her intuition told her that this man had something about him that was right for her. It is this inner sense of rightness that sustained Edna later in their relationship when Seymour left her to marry the other woman.

HOW DID YOUR RELATIONSHIP DEVELOP?

For the first eight months after their meeting, Edna and Seymour remained in their separate homes but saw each other almost every day. Neither stayed overnight in the other's home, as they both had teenagers. Still, they felt comfortable by frequently going into a bedroom, closing the door, and having sexual relations.

> * With this couple, even after their 16 years of being together, I could feel the sexual energy between them.

When in Chicago, visiting his niece, Seymour met a lady and rashly asked her to marry him. He returned and told Edna who was surprised and hurt. Seymour sold his house and loaded his personal items into a rental truck. Edna, caring for Seymour as a friend, loyally volunteered to drive with him. For a month they had no contact, but Edna still had faith that Seymour would return.

Their relationship should have ceased when Seymour married. But as Edna, a believer in astrological forecasts, stated, "From the beginning, our astrological signs and our personalities seemed to match well, and I strongly felt that ultimately, our futures were destined to be together."

> * Edna's strong faith that the relationship would work out may seem strange, but her conviction and instinct helped her rise above Seymour's sudden actions.

It's not unusual for a man who has been married for many years to impulsively jump into an unwise relationship after the death of a spouse. Edna understood this. Shortly after his hasty marriage, Seymour realized that it was not working out. He discovered that his wife was an alcoholic, and they had frequent bitter arguments. He had his own brand of patience; he did not want to hurt this women and decided not to leave her until she said that she wanted to end the marriage. Finally, she said she wanted out. Meanwhile, unhappy with his poor choice, he contacted Edna.

Edna told me, "Within a month, on my birthday, I received beautiful roses with a note—'with love, Seymour'—a lovely thought. Shortly thereafter, he started to phone me every Sunday. My Tarot cards told me he would return in January. After six months, Seymour divorced his wife, returned in January, and moved into my house." Edna's patience and her belief that she and Seymour were meant to be together, were justified at last.

Edna had an exceptional lack of rancor and ability to let Seymour find his own path. After he returned, his daughter said to her, "I'm surprised you took him back after what he did to you."

She replied, "He didn't do anything to me. If you let birds fly freely they return to the nest."

Edna and Seymour lived together five years before they married. The first four years were in Edna's home. The last year they purchased the retirement-community condominium where they now reside. During this time, Seymour never directly told Edna that he loved her. He called her "darling," and as Edna said, "He showed his affection for me with his eyes."

> * Here again, Edna was patient. She often noticed tears in Seymour's eyes and assumed that he needed time to grieve before committing himself to her. Without pressuring him, she waited.

Then one day, while shopping together in a large department store, at the top of a flight of stairs, Seymour paused, looked directly at Edna, and said he loved her, asking, "Will you marry me?" They were married shortly thereafter by a judge, on a date that astrological signs pointed to as propitious.

WHAT WERE YOUR EARLY LIVES LIKE?

Edna

Edna was the oldest of three sisters. Her parent's marriage was an unhappy one. Her father, an alcoholic, often would spank the children when drunk, but in spite of that, she felt a closeness to him. Her mother would force the children to go into the field to cut switches. Then she would beat them with the switches until they stopped screaming. As a young woman, despite the fact that her mother abused her and often asked her to leave, Edna stayed home, worked, and helped support the family.

> * Even as a young adult, Edna was patient in seeking love, but her longed-for closeness with her mother never occurred. Fortunately, her patience with Seymour won her a good relationship with a man who truly loves her.

Seymour

Seymour was raised in an orthodox Jewish family. His parents were both immigrants from Europe. He had one sister, five years younger. His father, a doctor, worked as a milkman to support the family during the Depression. Seymour describes his childhood as a happy one. He was especially close to his father, who took him to ball games and movies. His sister married an Israeli, moved to Israel, and still resides there. Seymour feels a strong allegiance to that country and has visited Israel several times with Edna.

WHAT WERE YOUR PREVIOUS RELATIONSHIPS LIKE?

Edna

Edna married her first husband when she was 23. During their 25 years of marriage, they had four children—two boys and two girls. Her husband was an insurance agent, and their income was erratic. Edna helped support the family by working on and off in various social work agencies. She and the children received little love or attention from her husband. He had a long extramarital affair, and Edna learned of it when this woman called the house. Although her husband broke off this affair, their marriage was still very strained. Edna felt unable to leave because of her concern for their four children. During this time she became depressed and often thought of killing herself.

To add a lighter note to this sad story, when Edna told me this, Seymour interjected, "Now there's many a day when she feels like killing me." Edna laughed and slapped him on the thigh.

Toward the end of her marriage, the whole family attended counseling. The counselor told Edna that her husband wanted a divorce. Sometime after he left home, she learned through a friend that he had had another long-term affair during their marriage.

> * Edna had a difficult childhood, that perhaps, led to her courting rejection again in her long and unhappy first marriage. A child mistreated by his or her parents may repeat the original trauma in an unsuccessful marriage, hoping in vain to receive from a mate the love never found as a child.
>
> With her first husband, Edna showed patience by staying with him 25 years despite much unhappiness. In retrospect, this might seem unwise, but with four

children, one does not leave a marriage lightly. Although her husband was the one who asked for the divorce, Edna was strong enough to leave him and make a good life for herself and the children.

The patience that Edna showed later in life with Seymour was of a different genre, and the results are much happier than those of her first marriage. Her sensitive awareness of the positive qualities in Seymour gave her the inner strength to be patient.

I find that often individuals working in helping professions, as Edna did as a social worker, have had childhoods difficult enough to make them sensitive to what is going on at a deeper level with others. If a child is going to be shouted at or hit by an erratic parent, she learns to be alert to that parent's every move. This sensitive antenna serves her well in later life by picking up both positive and negative "vibes"—a valuable ability, both professionally and personally. In her private life, Edna sensed Seymour's goodness and his love for her before he was ready to act upon it.

Seymour

Seymour was married to his first wife 37 years. They had three daughters. He had tears in his eyes as he spoke to me of her. He describes their marriage as a good one, but at the same time he told me she was strong willed, held grudges, and was responsible for a feud among his children that is ongoing.

* I suspect he loved his wife very much but understandably, has somewhat mixed feelings toward her. It is not unusual for grieving to be more difficult when feelings are

> ambivalent. The conflicting emotions are harder to accept, and the entire process may take longer to work through on either a conscious or an unconscious level.

Edna believes that it took Seymour five years to complete this grieving and be ready to propose marriage. Seymour, who is not as psychologically sophisticated as is Edna, only knows that for five years he had abnormally high blood pressure, which abated after his marriage to Edna.

> * Often, if an individual is not consciously aware of an emotion, this unrecognized feeling takes a bodily toll. In Seymour's case, his emotions may have been both sadness for the loss of his wife, whom he loved for her many good qualities, and anger at her for causing the rift among his children.

WHAT IS YOUR ONGOING RELATIONSHIP LIKE?

Edna and Seymour see themselves as "soul mates" and "mentally in tune." They often know what the other is thinking and feeling. Frequently they have the same thought at the same time and see each other as "mirror images of each other." Their marriage is filled with fun. They laugh, hug, and kiss a lot. A good part of their humor consists of teasing each other. At first, their children thought they were fighting, but now they realize that is just how this couple interacts.

After I finished interviewing Seymour, Edna entered the room. "I've just been telling her what a terrible wife you are," Seymour told her. Edna laughed and rubbed his back.

> * Humor is an important part of Edna and Seymour's relationship, as it is with many older couples. It buffers

conflict that may arise over habits previously formed. It can alleviate sadness that comes with declining health.

Teasing is a type of humor that can be hostile, but for Edna and Seymour, it is an indirect way of speaking of their love for each other, and it adds spice to their relationship. As Seymour told Edna after he proposed, "**when married, we'll never be bored**."

Edna and Seymour's joy in being together is augmented by their many activities. Edna makes and sells ceramics. Seymour collects and displays Indian arrowheads. Edna is also a photographer and displays her work. They play golf and workout in the community gym. They read and discuss the same books and have traveled extensively.

EDNA AND SEYMOUR'S ADVICE

Edna and Seymour offered some useful suggestions to other older persons who are forming new relationships. They stress acceptance of one's partner for who he or she is.

They say, "When two people get together, they have to explore their thoughts and feelings. This takes time and honesty. There are always differences, and you have to decide which ones you can accept. Some compromises and adjustments are necessary, but you really cannot expect another person to change his or her essential self. Too many people perceive what they think the other person wants and try to fill that role. You should continue to be who you are."

FINAL THOUGHTS

Edna showed unusual acceptance of Seymour's brief, unwise marriage and the time it took to grieve for his deceased wife before being fully committed to her. Seymour was accepting of Edna's beliefs in astrology and psychic phenomena. Their basic compatibility became the most important factor in their relationship.

It's very unusual for older couples, newly coupled, to have the experience of a partner leaving for another and then returning, but all must show patience in accepting differing beliefs and habits. It also takes patience and understanding to wait until your partner is fully committed. Often, after the death of a beloved spouse or a bitter divorce, one partner may take much longer that the other to open his or her heart in a new relationship.

Seymour and Edna tell us to first decide what you can live with and what's really important to you. If you then make the choice to be with someone, acceptance of that person as he or she is, is essential to a good relationship.

Chapter 10

(Interview: Karin and John)

"ARE YOU TWO IN LOVE? I SAW YOU HUGGING."

Karin and John taught Karin's six-year-old granddaughter to ride a bicycle. They were so delighted to see her confidently riding, they embraced each other. The granddaughter asked, "Are you two in love?

"Yes, why do you ask?" said Karin.

"Because I saw you hugging."

THEME
Respecting Different Needs for Closeness

Often the two individuals who make up a couple have different needs for closeness. John would like to live with Karin. She's much more cautious, and he is willing to wait. They recognize and respect these dissimilar needs in each other, and while continuing to live separately, they enjoy a loving relationship.

INTRODUCING KARIN AND JOHN

Karin's and John's residences are about a 20-minute drive apart. I visited John first. He rents a sparsely furnished apartment in a large city. John is an attractive man and looks much younger than his 69 years. He is tall, well built, with thinning reddish-gray hair and piercing blue eyes. He was intense and direct during our interview.

John retired from a career in county social service at the age of 50. After that, he earned additional income by managing several small businesses. He now teaches ballroom dancing several evenings a week. He has been twice divorced and has had several other long-term relationships.

Karin lives in a home in a nearby suburban community. Her home is very pleasant, sunny, spacious, and attractively furnished. Karin comes from Denmark. She is 65 years old, but looks younger, and is tall, blond, blue-eyed, and speaks with a slight accent. Karin was friendly, frank, and gracious during the interview.

Karin has been a widow for 13 years, and John is the first man she has been involved with since her husband's death. When I saw her, she had been retired for less than two weeks from a job as an office manager that she held for the past seven years. Toward the end of our interview, John came to her home and I saw them there together.

HOW DID YOU MEET?

Karin and John were both members of the same ballroom dance club. John was involved with another woman at the time but often danced with Karin. Each time he danced with her he would forget her name. "I have a thing about forgetting a woman's name, especially if I'm interested in her and I can't act on it." Karin eventually got annoyed with him and said, "If you don't want to remember my name, forget it." After that he remembered her name—forever.

After about a year, John broke up with his girlfriend, and then it took him a year to recover his good spirits. Finally, still attracted to Karin, and knowing that she was a hiker, he invited her to a club's lodge on the coast. Coincidentally, they were both members of the club. First she consented, but then she had second thoughts. "I can't sit in a car with him for two hours. He never talks." She called him and made an excuse not to go.

Several weekends later she went to the lodge with a girlfriend, and John was there with a friend. All four hiked together and had a great time. "Now I discovered that when we walk together, he doesn't stop talking!" Thus started their relationship.

WHAT ATTRACTED YOU TO EACH OTHER?

John expressed many reasons for finding Karin attractive. In fact, he was drawn to her before he was free to act upon it. He liked that she was in good physical condition, with a lot of energy. He recognized that she was down to earth, smiled easily, flirted, and had fun when she danced. He always has been attracted to somewhat different women and liked her Danish accent. "I love to look at her, love to dance with her, and love the way she talks." He was also attracted to her being a grandparent and very devoted to her grandchildren. At first he was concerned that she was overloading herself with this involvement but now realizes that "it's her nature."

> * John's initial concern about Karin's involvement with her grandchildren gradually faded. Perhaps he was a little jealous at first. As he got to know Karin and her grandchildren better, he became more secure, and his concern diminished. This kind of acceptance often comes naturally as a relationship develops.

Karin always thought she would like to get to know John, even when he was involved with another woman. She was attracted by his looks, the way he danced, and that he seemed to be a pleasant person.

She realizes that "looks come first, but they can lead to a disappointment." Obviously, that didn't happen in this relationship.

* There is more to looks than body build and facial features. Personality is expressed in the way one's body is held and moves. A smile, a facial expression, or the look in one's eyes, all shine through and give a message. Often this message is read on an unconscious level upon meeting a new person.

HOW DID YOUR RELATIONSHIP DEVELOP?

Very soon after the hiking weekend, John asked Karin to a concert and then to three social activities. Thinking he was rushing her, she accepted the concert, but refused the other invitations, saying, "I have to work."

* Right at the beginning, with his many invitations, John showed a greater need for closeness than did Karin.

John went on a trip for a week, and when he returned, he and Karin became closer and eventually became involved sexually. According to John, "I fell in love pretty fast—but not like I used to. Formerly, I'd fall in love with no questions. This time I used some judgment in my choice and waited for a go-ahead from the woman. I used to think I could change a woman who was rejecting me." Laughingly he continued, "I was so lovable, how could anyone resist me?"

In the summer Karin went for a long visit to Denmark, and on her return, she and John resumed their relationship. While Karin was still working, they spent weekends together, mostly at her home as it was larger, and they saw each other once or twice during the week for dancing. Since she has retired, John stays longer at her home, approximately four days a week. He keeps some clothes in the closet of her extra bedroom. They are planning a vacation of several weeks, their first vacation together.

WHAT WERE YOUR EARLY LIVES LIKE?

Karin

Karin was raised in a small, rural town in Denmark. She is the middle child, having an older brother and a younger sister. Her father was an accountant and died when she was 12 years old. She didn't get much affection from either parent but there was stability, and she knew she was loved.

> * In my experience, Scandinavian families are not especially affectionate, but there is much closeness. My late husband was of mixed Dutch and Norwegian ancestry. When I visit his family in Holland, I see little overt affection, but there is a discernible strong attachment among all family members.

Karin has many happy memories of her childhood. In the winter she skied to school and skated on the ponds. In the summer, along with her siblings, she picked berries, and they ate a lot of homegrown food from the family's garden. Now, as an adult, she is able to be affectionate with her mother, who is responsive to it. Her mother, in her 90s, is in failing health, and is in a rest home in Denmark. Karin phones her weekly and visits every year.

Karin left home to go to college on a scholarship. She graduated with a degree in languages and also attended business school. After finishing school, she continued to live on her own and worked in business.

John

John was raised in Southern California, the youngest of three children, with an older sister and brother. His father was a lawyer, and during his early childhood, the family was well off. When he was seven, his father died. John recalls his father as working long hours, but being warm and affectionate, playing with the children on weekends. His mother was ill with rheumatic fever for a year after her husband died, but when she recovered, she went to work as a telephone operator. She was always there for her children and had a good sense of humor, but her life was hard, and she wasn't affectionate. When the children didn't behave, she would threaten to send them to a home for wayward children. John described his relationship with his mother as one in which he was always trying to make her happy for fear he might be sent away. John believes this has much to do with his neediness and his desire to please the woman he is with.

> * I see desire to please in John's self-criticism and his worrying about traits that may not really bother Karin. His previous rushing into relationships and his present desire to live with Karin before she is ready may arise from early fears of abandonment.

On the positive side, John and his siblings were active in scouts, sports, and many other activities with friends. This continued into his adult life. Even now, at almost 70, he is still active physically and socially.

WHAT WERE YOUR PREVIOUS RELATIONSHIPS LIKE?

Karin

When Karin was 25, she met her 27-year-old husband to-be at a summer Quaker youth camp in Denmark. People from all over the world attended, and he was from the United States. She came to this country with him, and they were married here. The marriage lasted 27 years. They had two sons. Her husband was a chiropractor and she helped in his office. He died at age 54 of a lung disease caused by being exposed to asbestos while in the Navy. Karin had a long grieving period, but she was never depressed and was able to function, mainly because she could cry freely.

> * There is a real difference between grief and depression, and the outward expression of grief does much to dispel depression. I personally know the difference. I was in my forties when my brother died, and I was unable to cry. Outwardly I seemed okay, but for two years it felt like as though a pale gray screen stood between me and the world. When my husband died, I was 62 and alone in our home. Then when the waves of grief came over me, I was able to cry and yes, scream and howl. The grief was interspersed with periods of being able to enjoy life; thus I never felt that gray, grinding depression.

After her husband's death, Karin returned to school and attained another degree, this time in business administration. She enjoyed it, did very well, and this helped her self-confidence. She obtained an administrative position with a chiropractic society that lasted for seven years, until her retirement. Much like **Naomi**, who also experienced a lengthy first marriage, Karin enjoyed a period of being alone with increasing independence. If she felt lonely, she called a friend and shared activities. Unlike Naomi, she did not date, but neither women engaged in sexual activity until their present relationships.

> * For a woman like Karin or Naomi, who has been in a lengthy, traditional marriage, the period of widowhood brings a new experience of working and being in charge of her own life. She is no longer answerable to a husband or children and, once the initial grief is past, the new freedom is exhilarating. No wonder Karin is reluctant to give this up in exchange for the closeness of living with John.

I asked Karin if she noticed similarities between her deceased husband and John. "Yes—they are both a little quirky. That's the kind of person I like. Danes are very straight-laced, and I like unusual people." John, like her late husband, doesn't enjoy shopping for clothes; he likes to play jokes, and he is not overly concerned with money. Her husband grew a beard, biked to work, and did a lot of pro-bono service, so they never became wealthy. Thus, it doesn't bother her that John lives in a simple manner. "Though," she stated, "I wouldn't move into his place—it's too small."

> * Like **Gayle**, Karin is not concerned that her partner is less well off financially than herself. And should they eventually live together, John would share her house as **Jim** shares Gayle's home. It was easy for Jim to move in with Gayle, and John is not disturbed at the thought of leaving his small apartment. In fact, he partially lives in Karin's home now.

Karin feels free to talk to John about her husband and tells him some funny incidents from her marriage. John, in turn, has no difficulties talking about his previous relationships.

John

John married his first wife when he was 25 years old. This marriage lasted 20 years. They raised three boys and a girl. During this time, John worked as a county social worker. When the children became teenagers, his wife began to have difficulties with them, and engaged in severe arguments with one of the children. Rather than fight, John remained outwardly the model husband but distanced himself emotionally from his wife and family. "I had worked myself into a hole, playing the role of a good husband and father, and neglected to take care of myself. I felt I had to get out from under these burdens," he disclosed. "I had dreams that I would curl up and die if I didn't leave." He and his wife went unsuccessfully to family and couples' therapy. Then John attended a 10-week personal enrichment encounter (such groups were common in the '70s). "At the sessions, I had a taste of what it would be like to leave the marriage. I felt more life and energy." At age 44, John divorced his wife. He continued to see his children regularly and always paid for child support. He is now a committed grandparent.

From age 44 to 69, John had a number of relationships. His second marriage lasted 11 years. That wife was better off financially than he was. He moved into her house in a different community and worked in her business. After a number of years, she began to take trips without him, and he started to feel lonely and rejected. After several separations, they divorced.

Following his second marriage, John described another relationship that was fairly long lived. For five years he resided on and off with a woman with whom he had many conflicts. "It was a mess, and I should have ended it much sooner."

> * In his second marriage, John felt rejected, as he must have felt when his mother threatened to send him to a children's home. In his next long relationship, his reluctance to end it sooner might have come from these earlier insecurities.

John was involved in another fairly long relationship in which they did not live together. The lady was 12 years younger and had teenage boys. It did not work out. And, as might be expected of an attractive, socially active man, John had a number of other romances of shorter duration, one with the woman with whom he was associated when he first met Karin at the dance club.

> * John's ease in finding women substantiates the belief that it is easier for an older man to find a partner than it is for an older woman to do so. But finding a partner isn't enough. John's previous relationships did not work out well. It needs to be the right partner, and you need to be ready emotionally. (See Chapter 22 for information about being ready to find a partner.)

Because John obviously was hoping that he and Karin would go on together indefinitely, I asked him in what way she differed from others with whom he had been involved. He sees her as a much more secure and settled person than the other women in his life. The exception is his first wife, a stable woman, with whom he lived for 20 years. But unlike his first marriage, with Karin there are no problems of work or raising children. Also, more than in any other previous relationship, he and Karin are able to talk out their differences so that he is not left holding resentments.

TO LIVE OR NOT TO LIVE TOGETHER ... THAT IS THE QUESTION

Though Karin and John reside separately, they started talking about living together early in their relationship. The understanding is that John would move into Karin's larger, more comfortable home. It is John who is eager for them to live together. "I feel better, more secure, when living with someone," he said. At the same time, John is aware that he tends to be "emotionally needy" and is in psychotherapy to deal with this issue. As much as he wants to live with Karin, he doesn't want to rush into such an arrangement, as he did previously. Karin is hesitant and is in no hurry. Neither of them has made any mention of marriage.

> * Karin is afraid that living together would take away some of the romance between them. She likes not seeing John for a day or two and then looking forward to being with him. **Nancy**, who lives separately from **Pat**, also appreciates her time alone and believes that there is more romance between her and Pat when they do not see each other daily.

Karin wants any living together to be on a trial basis so that if it doesn't work out, John would not have lost his very desirable apartment. Karin is nervous about both of them being retired, having unstructured time, and thus getting on each other's nerves if they live together. She also is concerned about this extra time when living alone, and plans to take courses and serve as a volunteer.

* Unstructured time often is a concern as an individual is about to retire. I went through a brief period of high anxiety prior to my retirement from the agency where I had worked for many years. It did not take me long to structure my time; in fact, it became too full. I find this true of many active retirees and many of the couples interviewed. They wonder, as do I, how they ever fit in all they must do when working.

WHAT ARE YOUR ACTIVITIES AND INTERESTS?

Karin and John have many interests in common. They dance, walk, and bike together. John also runs regularly. They often play and fool around when they dance and have just learned the 1920s routine of "black bottom." They both love classical music, and Karin also likes folk music. Karin is an artist, and on her living room wall is a beautiful watercolor of a winter scene. They both enjoy going to the movies together (they have the same taste) and like discussing the film afterwards. John takes Tai Chi at a senior center, and now that she is retired, Karin plans to join him.

One thing that they definitely do not share is John's love of spectator sports. He watches sporting events a great deal on television and reads the sports section of the newspaper. If he reads details aloud to Karin, she says, "I'm not listening." Karin told me, "It's ironic. I've ended up with the same type of person as I had before. My husband loved horses. He rode, went to the races, and read about bets, odds, and race payoffs. I was never interested." With John this difference is no problem. Karin sometimes watches a game with John, knitting or reading, and is learning a little about baseball. Or, she just goes to another room and does something else.

* My opinion is that love of spectator sports is very much culturally determined. My own deceased husband, who, like Karin, was from Europe, had no interest in spectator sports, but now Jerry, a true American, is glued to professional football throughout the season.

WHAT ADJUSTMENTS HAVE YOU MADE?

Karin has a very positive outlook on this issue. "John is flexible ... very easy to be around. It's amazing, there are no adjustments. We just seem to flow. He helps with chores when asked. I'm a neatnick, but he's neat too." They both like the same food, near to vegetarianism, and often cook together. "He eats faster than I do, but my husband did too," she added, "I just ask him to slow down. It doesn't really bother me."

John tends to be self-critical and is concerned that he is four-and-a-half years older than Karin. He believes he has always had a poor memory, especially for names and places, and that it is getting worse now that he is older. He thinks that sometimes this annoys Karin. Also, because of being older, he worries that he naps during the day more than Karin does. John is tired after running or after many hours of dancing, and I believe he is just beginning to accept the fact that perhaps he can't do as much physically as formerly without some extra rest. He is pleased that Karin is starting to need naps too.

* It is good to keep physically active when older, but it is also necessary to accept with grace whatever natural slowing down occurs with age.

In terms of sleeping, they share the same bed, but John gets colder than Karin does. No problem. He just pulls the bedspread over himself.

FINAL THOUGHTS

For Karin and John, the question as to when, if ever, they will live together, is still unsettled. John's desire to live with Karin, possibly prematurely, comes from early insecurities. He is aware of this issue and is working on it in psychotherapy. Karin, after a long marriage in which she was a housewife, is reluctant to give up her newly found independence and is much more cautious about their living together.

These differing needs for closeness occur frequently in older couples in the early stages of a relationship. If both partners understand and respect each other's desires, there should be minimal conflict over this issue. Decisions about the future can be put aside, and then each partner can, as do Karin and John, entirely enjoy their full and happy new life together.

Chapter 11

(Interview: Joyce and Bill)

TROUBLE ... TROUBLE ... WILL IT LAST?

They started off with high hopes, having similar values in life, hiking together, becoming good friends, and then starting to live together. After a year, things gradually deteriorated. "Now we seem to be just biding our time to see what's going to happen between us."

THEME
Are Interests in Common Enough?

Despite many difficulties, Joyce and Bill are still together. They have a multitude of common interests—enjoying vacations together, hiking and camping, fine dining, and reading similar books. Bill's grandchildren are important to both of them. But is all this enough to make up for the power struggle in their daily lives and the resulting lack of tenderness and sexuality in their relationship?

INTRODUCING JOYCE AND BILL

Joyce is 64 years old, soft spoken, with brown hair and eyes that easily tear when discussing her relationship with Bill. Bill is 66 years of age, with a trim build, a gray mustache, and an outgoing, friendly manner. He is gregarious and talkative. She is a bit shy and more of a listener. They met three years ago and each is retired.

They live in Joyce's house in a small, rural community. Joyce does a lot of crocheting and knitting; she enjoys gardening and continues with her artwork. The house is reasonably neat but cluttered, containing many antiques and some valuable paintings that Bill brought with him. They have two pets—Bill's dog and Joyce's cat.

Joyce has a degree in art. For 30 years she was a teacher and still is active with her freelance art projects. Bill is a retired fireman and is now skilled at using a computer.

HOW DID YOU MEET?

Both Joyce and Bill belonged to the same hiking club. The club meets regularly in the mountains near Joyce's home, and she hiked with them regularly. Bill lived in a nearby city, and he joined them occasionally. On one outing Joyce and Bill walked together and engaged in animated conversation. They lunched together after the hike, and the attraction between them started to grow. As Bill said, "Our meeting took place at the right time for both of us."

HOW WERE YOU ATTRACTED TO EACH OTHER?

Shortly after they met, both Joyce and Bill recognized that they liked to do the same sorts of things, enjoying outdoor activities, being in the mountains, traveling, reading, and discussing the same books. Bill admired Joyce's youthfulness, her high level of physical activity, and her artistic competency. Joyce liked Bill's friendly, outgoing personality and was particularly attracted to his grandchildren, as she has none of her own.

HOW DID YOUR RELATIONSHIP DEVELOP?

After hiking and dining together a few times, Joyce and Bill's relationship developed rapidly. Bill visited with Joyce in her home, and she drove to his house, some 30 miles away. After four months, they became sexually involved. They then decided to live together in Joyce's country home and have resided there for the past two years. Bill sold his city home, as he was ready for a change and was happy to live in the country.

Early in their relationship, Joyce and Bill considered marriage, but as time passed, they decided it was not appropriate for them. For the first year together, they were both still working, and their life together was pleasant. They shared many activities and enjoyed their travels. Once they both retired, their time together increased, and their good relationship began to deteriorate.

> * Without work or children to raise, togetherness can be overwhelming for an older couple, newly coupled. People need to have a judicious combination of time together and time apart, and this will vary for each couple.

Joyce believed that Bill had difficulties adjusting to what she wanted in terms of housekeeping, daily routines, and changes from his previous life's activities. Bill still felt a strong attachment to his deceased wife, whom he believed understood him very well and knew how to deal with him, which Joyce did not. He felt controlled by Joyce and wanted more time to himself. These differences resulted in many quarrels, followed by long periods of withdrawal.

WHAT WERE YOUR PREVIOUS RELATIONSHIPS LIKE?

Joyce

Joyce had been married twice before, with her first marriage at age 21. They had two children, but her husband was not close to them, and Joyce had the primary responsibility of raising the children. Her husband had earned a comfortable income, but as Joyce said, "Money does not count if you don't get along together." They were divorced after 12 years. Her children are now in their 30s, and she has no grandchildren.

Joyce married again when she was 45 years old. This marriage also lasted for 12 years. As time went on, her second husband had a number of extramarital affairs, and Joyce again decided to terminate the marriage. She made a vow "not to get married again, but just hang in there and pursue my own life." When the second marriage ended, Joyce was 57 years old, and she was alone and independent for 7 years before meeting Bill.

Bill

Bill met his wife when he was 17 years old, and they were married when he was 28. The marriage lasted 38 years until his wife died of a sudden heart attack. There were tears in Bill's eyes when he spoke of his wife. In our discussion, he admitted that he has a temper and can be difficult at times. Bill said with fond remembrance, "My wife knew how to handle me."

* I wonder how she did "handle" him. Was she submissive? Did she just calmly ignore his temper? This "handling" seems to be difficult for Joyce.

Bill and his wife had two daughters, and now he has three grandchildren. After the death of his wife, one of his daughters, her husband and their son, moved into his house with him. His daughter, whom he believed was overly attached to him, became very possessive of the house, and this disturbed Bill. This was one factor that motivated Bill to sell the house and put some distance between himself and his children.

This daughter's relationship with Joyce is not very good, perhaps because of her attachment to her father. One daughter's 12-year-old daughter is very close to Joyce, and Joyce very much enjoys having the child visit them. Joyce is an artist, skilled in crafts and handwork, and devotes much time to teaching this young girl. I saw Bill's grandchild when I visited, and she was busily knitting a scarf.

* This relationship with Bill's grandchild is very important to Joyce, who has no grandchildren of her own. It is one factor that is holding Bill and Joyce's relationship together.

DIFFERENCES LEADING TO PROBLEMS

Bill and Joyce's relationship is not developing in the manner that either of them had hoped it would when they first became interested in each other. Their discussions with me were very frank. They each clearly revealed the problems they face.

Joyce and Bill's prior relationships affect their present adjustments. Bill was married 38 years and describes an exceptionally understanding wife. He told me, "My wife has a magnetic personality," using the present tense, although she had been dead for several years.

> * It seems that Bill has not emotionally separated himself from his wife. Many others interviewed held fond memories of their deceased spouses but were able to form new attachments. Bill seems to be idealizing his late wife and thus, not allowing himself to fully commit to Joyce.

In the seven years that Joyce has been living alone, she has been self-sufficient, living her life and arranging her home in ways that pleased her. This independence presents a problem for Bill, who sees Joyce as attempting to control him. Unfortunately, Joyce has had little practice in clearly stating what she wants in a manner that is not disturbing to Bill. Instead when angry, she withdraws her affection, which I believe Bill badly needs, and she holds on to hurts. When I saw them together, he refused to look at her.

> * To give Joyce credit, with the hurt and anger that Bill feels now, I don't know if he could actually hear her words and recognize her needs. It is not possible to listen clearly when emotionally upset.

Problems with health have added to this couple's difficulties. Joyce had knee surgery a year ago and therefore, hikes easier trails. This disturbs Bill, who wants her company and urges her to join him on more strenuous outings.

Bill can be irritable because of high blood pressure not adequately controlled. He has attended stress-management courses and is now a vegetarian. The blood pressure medication affects his sexual desire and performance.

When their sexual activity started, it was very satisfying and enjoyable for both of them. Bill had helped Joyce relax and become more sexually active, but because of their relationship problems and the effects of Bill's high blood-pressure medication, their intercourse has become limited and not satisfactory for either of them. As Joyce stated, "I feel it necessary to be deeply in love to have sexual fulfillment. Our present relationship does not support good sex."

> * Concerning a couple's sexual life, it is a question of which comes first, "the chicken or the egg." If you are angry and hurt, sex usually is not satisfactory, but the good feelings from enjoyable sex affect daily life, making differences seem much less important.

Financial arrangements are not a problem. Bill and Joyce deposit an equal amount of money from their monthly retirement incomes into a joint checking account to pay for food, house expenses, and taxes. Each one also has a separate account to cover other costs. Bill insists on paying the full amount for travel, dining out, and other entertainment.

> * Traditionally, the man pays for such expenses. Living in Joyce's home must be difficult for Bill, as it means fitting into another person's lifestyle. **John**, who spends much of his time in **Karin's** home, also insists on paying for all entertainment, and doing so must help both men's self-esteem.

Both Joyce and Bill have established separate Living Trusts for each one's assets to go to their own children. Bill is considering putting aside a small percentage of his investments for Joyce if he should die first.

> * It is encouraging that despite their differences, they handle their expenses cooperatively, and that Bill wants to help Joyce with her future financial security.

WHAT ARE YOUR THOUGHTS ABOUT YOUR RELATIONSHIP?

During their separate interviews, Joyce and Bill both stated the same two wishes—wanting a close friend and not wanting to live alone. They expressed their positions from both negative and positive viewpoints and made many statements that indicate the difficulties they face and their ambivalence.

Negative Comments from Joyce

"I have had lots of arguments in my life, and I don't mean to argue now. When we start to argue, I retreat and leave the room."

* She doesn't come back to face the issue with Bill at a calmer time.

"We did not realize our differences before starting to live together."

* There are always differences when people live together, especially with older couples who have had a variety of experiences. They must know how to work out those differences.

"Things were much better before living together. Now it's like a marriage."

* Her experience with previous marriages was poor.

"He likes to control people, and if he doesn't get his way, he's upset, but I won't let him dominate me."

* Bill in turn, feels Joyce tries to dominate him. They are in a battle for control, as are many couples with problems.

"Our present relationship doesn't support good sex."

* How true.

"I would like him to be more affectionate."

* He might like affection also. Sometimes it helps to give affection first when you want it from your partner, but you must feel good about the other person to do so.

"When he gets mad, he makes me sit down and he lectures to me. I get up and leave the room."

* Okay, but come back and talk it over later. Let him know you hate being lectured to.

"I am resigned to a relationship of convenience for both of us that is not passionate or sexual."

* So sad. Many couples are resigned this way.

"He doesn't know the feelings inside me."

* Could she, with help, tell him, and could he listen?

"He says he's trapped, but he can leave any time he wants to."

* Does she really want him to leave? Bill has said she'd have to throw him out, and if she wanted to, she could.

Negative Comments from Bill

"I do not want to be owned or dominated."

* They are in a control battle. Bill is living in Joyce's house, which makes it particularly difficult for him.

"I need an escape hatch … I could take my dog and camp in the wilderness. But if I do, it may automatically be taken that I've given up and am walking out."

* Is there a positive way he can tell her of his need for space?

"I will not get married again."

* Does he mean that he is reluctant to fully commit himself? Recall that he still feels attached to his late wife.

"Sometimes I am treated as a second grader."

* This may possibly be true.

"I'm not comfortable talking with Joyce about my deceased wife."

* I think the degree to which he still cares for and idealizes his wife would be difficult for Joyce to hear.

"It seems that the more familiar we get with each other, the worse it gets between us."

* Are they losing respect for each other?

"There are some rough edges in our relationship with some things being taken the wrong way and I don't know how to solve it."

* This indicates a desire to make things better. See the list of positive comments by both of them starting shortly.

"I miss her when she's not here, but I won't be owned or dominated by her."

* Ambivalence and the control issue.

"At times it's not worth the effort to be affectionate, and I know she thrives on affection."

* Does he need affection also?

"I don't know what the solution is. I like her and I like it here."

* Does he let her know he likes her, and would "like" rather than "love" be enough for Joyce?

"I don't want to leave unless she throws me out."

* Here he wants her to take the responsibility for ending their relationship.

Among their negative statements are some positive ones that show potential for holding this relationship together and starting the all-important healing process.

Positive Comments from Joyce

"I know he really tries to be good."
"Down the road we'll get back together."
"We should not break up, it's too hard on the grandchildren."

* An interesting twist on the reason younger couples use to stay together—for the sake of their children rather than grandchildren.

"When we have problems, we should sit down and talk—map out our goals and decide together what to do to overcome the problem."

"We need to have understandings and make compromises."

"I don't think arguments are settled when people argue hot and heavy. It's a waste of energy. Life is too short."

"I want a loving relationship for the rest of my life."

Positive Comments from Bill

"Neither one of us wants to live alone."
"I am pleased when she is happy with herself."
"She's so talented and I love to see her artwork."
"We could live together as good friends and companions."

* Just "friends?" What about affection and sex?

"I really think enough of her to contribute to her financial security."

"I want someone to talk to and be playful with."

"I hope a good relationship between us can last forever."

"We should enjoy what we have—and sometimes we do!"

* I particularly like the last statement, "We should enjoy what we have—and sometimes we do!" My experience has been that couples with problems often fail to notice the times when they do get along well. Here Bill acknowledges that sometimes they do enjoy each other. Perhaps it is more often than either of them is aware of. I often give couples whom I am counseling an assignment to write down the good times they notice. The number of good interactions often is surprising to them.

POSTSCRIPT

I recently recontacted Joyce and Bill, and was delighted to learn that, though there are still difficulties, their time together is now more pleasant. Joyce has been very supportive and persistent in helping Bill find a physician who is able to prescribe the proper medication for his problem with high blood pressure. His blood pressure is under control, and he is much less irritable. Joyce in turn, is more understanding, as she realizes that there were tangible physiological reasons for Bill's crankiness. Many of the problems described in this chapter still exist, but Joyce and Bill have an increased respect for the role that medical conditions play in the quality of their day-to-day interactions.

FINAL THOUGHTS

I see Joyce and Bill as two good people, both hurting and in pain. The good news in the postscript has increased my hope for the success of their relationship. Are their troubles over? I doubt it. When there is a difficult history, the hurt and anger can linger. New skills are needed in communication and problem solving. They need to learn to listen to each other, not to store old hurts, and to express openly what they do appreciate. Then gradually, as negative encounters decrease, there will be more space for positive experiences filled with sharing, fun, affection, and enhanced sexuality.

To their credit, Joyce and Bill certainly have hung together through hard times. Neither ever seriously considered ending their relationship, and they never separated, even after a heated argument and a consequent period of withdrawal. This shows a genuine commitment to each other. Perhaps they eventually will be able to look back on these first few years together, knowing that by working on both their physiological and interpersonal problems, despite much **trouble ... trouble ... their union is lasting**.

Chapter 12

(Interview: Mary and Fred))

IT WAS MEANT TO BE

Imagine being young and single. You are at a party and find yourself attracted to someone who is married and not available. And then 35 years later, you meet that same person again and knowing "this is it." That happened to Fred, who now has been happily married to Mary for more than 20 years. Here is their story.

THEME
Reigniting the Spark

> Theories abound concerning what chemistry draws people together. Mary and Fred are evidence that a spark can be reignited after many years of no contact. There must be an awareness, even after 35 years, that something "fits." Given the right circumstances and a little luck, this chemistry can lead to a lasting relationship.

INTRODUCING MARY AND FRED

Mary is 85 years of age and Fred is 79, six years younger. They became reacquainted 23 years ago, when Mary was 62 and Fred was 56. At the time of their interview, they had been married 22 years. They are one of the oldest couples I've talked with. Like **Gayle** and **Jim**, the woman is older than the man. Fred is retired from a career in the Navy, where he served as a Commander and Mary spent the majority of her years as a housewife.

They greeted me warmly at the door of their small apartment, located in an elegant congregate living residence. Here lunch and dinner are provided, as well as housekeeping, transportation, and a large variety of activities. The three of us sat together around the kitchen table as we conversed. Mary was the more talkative, while Fred interspersed comments in a quiet, reflective manner. He is of medium build with slightly thinning gray hair. Mary is short, with soft silver hair, sparkling brown eyes, and a lively smile. She is slightly heavy. As she confided, "You can easily gain weight here."

> * It is understandable that a costly retirement facility would serve meals with several courses, including attractive desserts. While dietary requirements and preferences are accommodated, many delicious dishes tempt the residents. Most older folks who cook for themselves would not eat the quantity of food provided in this setting. With aging, metabolism slows down, and people are more sedentary. Under such circumstances, a great deal of self-control is needed to avoid weight gain.

HOW DID YOU MEET?

In 1940, at a social gathering held by his best friend, Fred met a young woman. At the time he was 20 and she was 26. His mind was on completing his college degree and then entering military service. Even though she was married, she impressed Fred as someone he would have liked to see again.

Then, 35 years later, Fred attended the eightieth birthday party for the father of another friend. Again he was introduced to a lady and had the feeling he had met her sometime previously. "Who was she?" he asked himself. Suddenly it came to him—this was the same person, now a widow, who had long ago so impressed him. "Oh, this is great!" Fred thought.

Mary remembered the two incidents in similar ways. When she met Fred the second time, she felt, "This is it!"

* Two of the other couples interviewed, **Ruth** and **Paul** and **Barbara** and **Leonard**, knew each other in work situations, felt an attraction to each other, but didn't act on it because one or both were already married. Years later they met again, and that same attraction was still there.

Both of these couples' early acquaintanceships were formed over a period of time, while Mary and Fred had met for the first time only briefly at a party. But they all must have known on some level that the qualities that had attracted them to each other many years ago, were still there.

There's an unconscious awareness that another's personality dovetails with yours. Mary is soft, feminine, and somewhat submissive, as are many women of her age bracket. Fred is a strong, straight-arrow man, as fits his previous occupation in the military. They complement each other.

This unconscious fit is not always healthy. For years as a young woman, I was attracted to brilliant, handsome, unstable men, much like my older brother, who I adored. Sometimes they left me brokenhearted, and sometimes I had enough sense to break off the relationship. My late husband, whom I married at the more emotionally mature age of 28, reminded me of my very loving, reliable father, and the marriage was a good one. Mary and Fred were mature enough that the chemistry between them led to a good and lasting relationship.

HOW WERE YOU ATTRACTED TO EACH OTHER?

What interested Fred in Mary? First, the remembrance of their first meeting many years ago had stayed in his memory. Now, at the second meeting, Fred felt good "vibes." To him, as a first impression, Mary offered an attractive appearance and was a good conversationalist.

Mary, when meeting Fred that second time, saw him as good looking and nicely dressed. After being a widow for seven years, she had the feeling that good fortune was smiling upon her.

* Neither Mary nor Fred was particularly articulate about what attracted each to the other. There must have been more than good looks and interesting conversation. Fred's statement about vibes makes the most sense to me. Vibes would explain an unconscious attraction that neither fully understood.

HOW DID YOUR RELATIONSHIP DEVELOP?

Their second meeting at the birthday party took place in the area where Mary resided. Fred lived a day's driving distance away. One week later, he phoned Mary to express his interest in her. They corresponded and spoke to each other twice a week on the telephone. A short while later, Fred traveled to see her. Then Mary visited his home, and their relationship strengthened.

Mary thought she might be considered "old fashioned," as her moral code decreed "no living together before marriage." Both she and Fred wanted to get to know each other better, so they waited until eight months after their second meeting to marry.

WHAT WERE YOUR PREVIOUS RELATIONSHIPS LIKE?

Mary

Mary was married when she was 16 years old to a 21-year-old carpenter. Her marriage was a good one that lasted 40 years. She has one son and now three grandchildren. Mary cashiered in a department store for seven years but stayed at home most of the time, being a homemaker and raising her son. Her husband died suddenly of a heart attack, and she was then a widow for seven years before meeting Fred.

Fred

Fred is now in his third marriage. The first one, during the war, was very unsatisfactory. That wife was a nurse and suddenly disappeared. Apparently, she had been using drugs and became quite unstable. They had one son, who was raised by Fred's mother.

Fred married again after the war. This second wife died of cancer 17 years later. They had no children. Fred now has a grandchild and two great grandchildren from his one son. Both Mary's and Fred's sons and their children accept their marriage.

WHAT ARE YOUR PRESENT LIVING ARRANGEMENTS LIKE?

When Mary and Fred married, they decided to live in Fred's expansive house. It was on an acre of land with many large windows that provided a magnificent view of the ocean. Mary left much behind, including her daughter and many friends. They lived in Fred's house for 10 years, and it took her some time to feel comfortable with new acquaintances in that area.

Fred's cousin was living in a retirement community, and they liked the idea. First however, they sold Fred's house and moved into a nearby condominium for 10 years. Then, two-and-a-half years ago, they decided to move back to the area where Mary had lived previously and purchased their present residence in the congregate living facility.

"These moves haven't been easy for me," said Mary. "I'm a people person, and I like to have good, close friends, but I'm a little shy. It took me some years to have a circle of friends and then, just when I felt at home, we moved. I like it where we are now, and I hope we stay put."

* Where to live is an important decision for many older couples. When one person moves into the partner's home, that individual will have the majority of adjustments to make—leaving friends, getting used to new surroundings and a new community, adjusting to the partner's standards and expectations in the home, and often parting with many of his or her own furnishings and other possessions. The homeowner also needs to make accommodations to the habits and desires of the new partner.

Often, selling both homes and moving to a new residence is the best plan. The key emotional advantage for moving into a new home together is that it can become "our home" for the couple.

WHAT PROBLEMS WERE FACED AND WHAT ADJUSTMENTS WERE MADE?

Even after 22 years of marriage, Mary and Fred are still adjusting to each other, as are most couples throughout the course of their relationship. They are able to laugh at their disagreements.

"I'm a neatnick," said Fred, "and I'm always picking up after Mary and putting things in their right place."

She made a face at him. "And," said Mary, as she put her arm on Fred's shoulder, "during a bingo game, this man will shout out as loud as can be, 'Be quiet and pay attention.' It's embarrassing." Fred believes that this behavior is a carry-over from his military experiences and might also be necessary because many older folks are hard of hearing.

Fred is on numerous mailing lists, and as a result, receives large quantities of advertisements, circulars, and other types of junk mail. He spends a great amount of time sitting and carefully reading his mail. This behavior angers Mary, who tells him he is very foolish and should stop it. In return, Fred gets annoyed, doesn't listen to her, and usually goes ahead with his reading. Mary concludes, "This is a common practice of men, and I won't fight it."

> * To "not fight it" Mary needs to accept this habit of Fred's and say nothing when he is perusing junk mail.

Mary believes that her first husband, and now Fred, have been over-protective of her. Her first husband did not want her to work outside their home. Now Fred watches her drinking of hard liquor, stating that he doesn't want her to imbibe more than she should. "And I only take one or two drinks a week. He shouldn't be concerned," interjects Mary.

At times, Mary wants some privacy and freedom from doing things together with Fred.

> * Actually, the retirement community offers many activities that Mary could attend without her husband, but the attitude of the times in which she was raised, makes this difficult for her. Remember, she is 85 years old now and

was married 40 years, starting at age 16. That was from 1930 to 1953. I assume that, like almost all women of that era, she did not enjoy much independence from her husband and family.

Perhaps the reason Mary does not act now on her stated desire to have more privacy and freedom is that, in the past, she had not often experienced independent activities. Thus, initiating such activities now could be difficult for her; but her desire to do so, and her belief that both husbands have been over-protective, demonstrates that, in some ways, her attitude is changing with the times.

WHAT ARE YOUR PRESENT ACTIVITIES?

Mary and Fred enjoy many activities together, most of which are provided by their community association. A bus takes them shopping, to restaurants, to the movies. This really suits Mary, who never learned to drive and never wanted to do so. In their facility, they take classes in history and Bible study. They also attend an exercise class together. On their own, they take tours, once or twice as year to many places out of the country. "We really do have fun together," said Fred, "and we'll keep traveling as long as we're physically able."

FINAL THOUGHTS

It is inspiring to know that a spark between two young people can be reignited after 35 years and that it can lead to more than 22 years of a happy marriage. As Mary says, "If you trust your own intuition and the chemistry's right, it doesn't matter how old you are—just do it."

Being older and in a different time of life might have helped the success of this union. Mary and Fred agree that a marriage can be a struggle when young. In a later marriage, being more secure financially and with children raised, a couple can have fewer worries and can concentrate on enjoying their lives together. For them, the coincidence of their meeting twice, twice being attracted to each other, and the second time both being free to form a relationship, proves beyond doubt that "**it was meant to be.**"

Chapter 13

(Interview: Carol and Ron)

AN UNUSUAL RELATIONSHIP ... MARRIED AND LIVING SEPARATELY

Carol: "We are cosmically connected ... drawn together by the forces."

Ron: "And we stuck together ... even through the worst of times. Even when we separated, our commitment was unbroken."

Opposites attract each other, although in this case it is difficult for them to live together. While facing one challenge after another, there remains a strong bond of love and support between them. Though the lifestyles and beliefs of Carol and Ron may differ from those of some readers, their problems and struggles are similar to many that older couples encounter. Therefore, reading of their strengths and adjustments can be most helpful.

THEME
A Third Option

Most couples having the amount of conflict that Carol and Ron experienced when they lived together would have ended their relationship. Yet some couples choose to remain living together, no matter what. Carol and Ron exemplify a third option. They are a loyal and loving married couple who live next door to each other.

INTRODUCING CAROL AND RON

Carol greeted me graciously at the entrance to her home. We walked though her house to the deck and held the interview there. Carol, age 64, a retired insurance broker, tall and slim, was casually dressed in a sweatshirt and pants. During much of this interview, she sat with legs crossed and her feet tucked under her in a lotus position. Her home, overlooking a garden, provides a feeling of quiet serenity. On the wall hang abstract paintings that Carol has created, and in her bedroom is a small altar she uses for meditation. Her cat sat curled at her feet while we talked.

The following day, I visited Ron, age 82. He is somewhat shorter than Carol, with a youthful-appearing, trim body. Ron is an aeronautical engineer, retired from his own consulting business. His house is a short distance from Carol's. It is very open, with large windows that bring in much light. Many plants are placed throughout the house, and I noticed a Buddha statue in the living room. Outside are two birdbaths and a large flagstone patio covered by a widely spreading oak tree.

HOW DID YOU MEET?

Both Carol and Ron enjoy mountain hiking and camping. When Carol was age 47 and Ron was 65, they were participants in a summer pack trip in the high Sierras. The custom for the trip was that as it neared its end, the group would celebrate with a champagne party. That afternoon a heavy rainstorm hit the camp and continued into the night. This did not stop the champagne from flowing. However, rain flooded Carol's tent, causing her to be cold and wet when, after the party, she attempted to sleep. For comfort, what should she do?

Carol is a strong feminist and has liberal political opinions. Although she saw Ron as somewhat of an "opinionated redneck," she desperately needed to be dry and warm. Since Ron was alone in a nearby tent, his place seemed to be the answer. She entered and, seeing her predicament, he invited her into his dry sleeping bag. Since her clothes were wet, she removed them all and joined him in the sleeping bag. Thus they spent the night together, keeping each other warm, but, as pointed out by both of them, with no sexual activity between them.

During the night, Carol reached over, pulling a blanket over Ron. As Ron observed, "this thoughtful gesture turned the tide for me." Then in the morning, Ron, in a sweet way, brought coffee to her. In describing this action to me, Carol's words were, "This shifted my feelings for him. Juices started flowing."

> * From the very start, they each expressed a loving consideration for each other, and it was this nurturing quality that each so much appreciated throughout their relationship.

They spent much of the next day together, joking and chasing each other like kids. Carol, from her perspective, summarized her feelings for Ron, "I was in love with him—absolutely gone—emotionally deep."

HOW WERE YOU ATTRACTED TO EACH OTHER?

Carol had a difficult childhood without a father. When she met Ron, she saw him as a strong, take-charge, caring person. Although she was, and still is, strong willed, Ron triggered her need for a father figure. She felt at the time, "Daddy will take care of everything."

* This need for a father figure is often the unconscious motivation for a woman to marry a much older man.

Ron had these answers to the "how were you attracted" question: "I was fascinated by her. She was different from any woman I ever met. She was totally uninhibited in her actions. This intrigued me. Falling in love with her was so refreshing."

HOW DID YOUR RELATIONSHIP DEVELOP?

After the end of the pack trip, in spite of the feelings they had for each other, they didn't plan to meet again soon. But a short time later, Carol had severe back pain and, recalling how helpful Ron had been to her in the mountains, she found his number and phoned him. He promised to bring her a "very effective" painkiller (which turned out to be Motrin™, available in any drugstore!).

Although at this time, Ron was still married to his first wife, they had been separated for two years and their divorce was forthcoming. He drove from his home in a small town to Carol's city residence and stayed overnight. Their sexual activity now started, and they frequently visited back and forth on weekends. As Carol said, "I have not looked at another man since. We became blissfully inseparable with lots of love between us."

They skied, hiked, motorcycled, and traveled together. Remembering these times, Ron observed, "She was such an energetic, alive person who liked exploring new things and taking chances. I found her so stimulating to be with."

Five years into their relationship, Ron approached Carol in a serious manner, saying "I think we should get married." At that time, Carol saw no reason of her own to marry.

"But I knew," noted Ron, "that a marriage license was the only way to protect her financially."

Carol smiled, "So I said okay."

* Here again, we see Ron's nurturing quality. He was better off financially than Carol and wanted to take care of her in the future.

They chose to marry after a silent retreat in a yoga ashram. For 10 days, no one spoke. When the silence ended, all the participants gathered in a large circle. Carol spoke first to Ron, "You had ten days to think, and I'm wondering if you've changed your mind about our wedding tomorrow."

Ron said nothing for a long, long time and everyone held their breath. Finally, he simply said, "You couldn't keep me from it." They were married the next day at the ashram.

WHAT PROBLEMS WERE FACED AND WHAT ADJUSTMENTS WERE MADE?

Eight years after their marriage, they sold their separate houses, and together bought a home in the city where Carol resided. They lived in this home for five years. At first all went well between them, but then things began to change. As Carol expressed it, "It became difficult for us to live together. We had one challenge after another between us. I learned that Ron is extremely compulsive and goal oriented. He is *not* a negotiator. Do it *his* way or not at all! He is used to doing things for himself—without asking or telling anyone. He'd put my things away because he is very neat, and then often I couldn't find them. It was extremely difficult for both of us. But when my painful back problem arose, he was very kind and supportive by shopping, cooking, and doing the laundry for both of us. But we did often argue and had verbal fights. We would become very angry, yell and scream, and call each other names".

* As it was for Carol and Ron, it often takes a period of time living together before differences between a couple become evident and disturbing. Cursing and name calling can lead to deep hurts and resentments. Carol and Ron were very aware of this danger, and to preserve their relationship, they decided to live separately.

"While there was still a strong attachment between us," Carol continued, "we had to get away from each other. We were not addressing our differences head-on. I bought a home at the coast, and we each entered psychotherapy to help with our disagreements. I sold my insurance business, and Ron came out to my coastal home and tried to live with me. He didn't like people in the town and could not accept living there. He truly was miserable. After eight months I asked him to leave, and we began to live separately."

* The town Carol was living in at that time was and still is a "hippie haven." She was very comfortable in that atmosphere and made many friends there. To Ron, the general ambiance of that town was extremely distasteful.

Ron agreed with Carol's reasons for their separation and added, "We still had different habits that were difficult to give up. She's fussy and more orderly that I am."

* It is interesting that both Carol and Ron describe each other as overly orderly, seeing this as a problem. People are orderly in different areas of their lives. For Jerry, it is important to turn off lights and keep detailed accounts of expenses. I am careful to put away papers and magazines and to maintain a clean house.

Despite their difficulties in living together, Carol and Ron continued their close relationship. Ron rented an apartment in a nearby city and often talked with Carol on the telephone. They would get together about three times a month. They still had strong affectionate feelings for each other.

After five years of living near Carol's coastal home, Ron decided that he preferred the country and moved to a small house on property he owned in a rural area. Then, wanting a larger house, he purchased one in a nearby suburban subdivision. Shortly thereafter, on his birthday, Carol came to visit. This new house needed a great deal of renovation before Ron would feel comfortable enough to move in. During her visit, he asked Carol if she would make changes in the house "as she'd like it to be." She warmly agreed to do this.

It took two months for workmen to renovate and improve the house. During this period, Carol lived in the house to supervise the construction, and Ron stayed in the small house that he still owns. They talked at length about their differences and the pain each one had caused the other. While they forgave each other, many disagreements continued. When the house was finished, Ron moved into his attractive, newly rebuilt home. Carol still thought that she could not live with him but wanted to be nearby. She sold her coastal home and bought a place in the same subdivision. Thus, they are now living just a few steps away from each other in the two homes that I visited during my interviews.

WHAT HAVE YOUR EARLY LIVES BEEN LIKE?

Carol

Carol's mother died shortly after she was born. Then her father abandoned her, leaving it up to his parents to raise her. Her grandparents lived on a farm in the Midwest. She was often alone, as her grandparents and their hired men were busy working on the farm. She roamed the fields by herself, unprotected. Her grandmother was very strict and controlling, and Carol, strong-willed even as a child, was sassy. Her grandmother often whipped her and washed her mouth out with soap. At an early age, she took up smoking and drinking. Her drinking became serious and continued even through the early part of her marriage to Ron. (Ron and Carol do not drink alcoholic beverages at all now.) Despite her problem with alcohol, Carol was successful in the work world, first as a secretary and bookkeeper, and then, after taking the necessary courses, by establishing her own insurance brokerage firm.

Ron

Ron was raised as an only child on a Texas ranch. As a youth, he was brought up by his mother after his father died. Independent and self-sufficient, he milked cows, and worked at the fountain in a soda shop while in high school. At age 12 he learned to fly an airplane. As a young man Ron completed a college degree in aeronautical engineering. Before World War II, he worked for a defense contractor but left for military service where he was trained as a bomber pilot, and later he engaged in extensive combat. After the war, he established his own successful consulting practice, which he sold shortly before meeting Carol.

WHAT WERE YOUR PREVIOUS RELATIONSHIPS LIKE?

Carol

At age 16, Carol married a 25-year-old man, mainly to leave the rural Midwest that she found suffocating. He was a hard-working, nice person. At that time, she had not completed high school, and he did not want her to return to school. School was important to Carol, and she did not like being controlled as she had been by her grandmother. She left her husband, and shortly thereafter they divorced.

A year later she married again. This marriage lasted for six years with drinking and verbal fighting. The result was another divorce.

Carol was then single until age 28, when she married for a third time. This husband decided to pursue a college degree while Carol worked long hours in an office. The two had little time together and her drinking continued. After seven years, they were divorced.

> * It is interesting that on three occasions, Carol dissolved a marriage, but the bond she and Ron formed has lasted despite many difficulties.

Considering her former marriages, Carol sincerely told me, "I could just walk away from them with no problem, but with Ron it's different. I'm totally committed to him and now, at his age, would never leave."

Ron

During the war, at age 22, Ron married and had one daughter. He and his wife had little in common and divorced when Ron was in his mid-30s. Then, three years later, they remarried for the sake of their daughter. They stayed together 28 years, but as Ron stated, "It became a dead marriage." They divorced again.

WHAT ARE YOUR PRESENT LIVES LIKE?

In the early years of Carol and Ron's relationship, they "partied" and drank a great deal. "But our health problems led us to turn our lives around," said Ron.

"I had a terribly painful problem with my back," continued Carol. "My spinal discs were degenerating. I was told I would eventually be crippled and be unable to walk. Ron even had to help me dress."

Ron stated, "And I developed cancer of the prostate about the time we married. I did have an orchiectomy (removal of the testosterone-forming glands that spread the cancer), but in addition to regular medical treatments, we wanted to do all we could on our own to overcome our physical problems."

"So," added Carol, "we went together to a yoga-based, vegetarian cancer retreat."

"And that started our journey," continued Ron. "We are still on it, and our health has improved markedly.

Ron and Carol now are vegetarians and grow vegetables and fruits in their respective gardens. Together they attend many retreats where they fast and meditate. Carol has studied to become a yoga instructor, teaches a class locally, and gives Ron yoga instruction every Saturday. Remarkably, as the result of their alternative healing activities, Carol no longer suffers with severe back problems. She is able to be physically active and takes daily four-mile walks. Sometimes Ron walks with her, and then she slows her pace to accommodate him.

Since Ron is now more than 80 years of age, they recognize the need to view life in a different perspective from when he was in his 60s. At that time, despite the chronological age difference of 18 years, Carol believed Ron was younger than she, both physically and mentally. Carol recalled that in those days, a few times she was asked for her senior identification, while Ron was considered to be too young! But now, they agree that he definitely has a slower pace of life. As Carol stated, "I'm ready to take a lengthy trip, but Ron doesn't want to think about it. It's partly his personality and, to a large degree, his advanced age."

* As an individual reaches about 80, there often is a slowing down and this can be hard for both partners to accept. It is easier if the one slowing down can accept the other person doing things without him or her. Ron accepts Carol's traveling, visiting with friends, and engaging in many other activities alone.

When a younger woman marries a much older man, as Carol did, she needs to look to the future and know that at a later date, she might have a much-less-active partner. If she has her own activities and interests, the adjustment will be much less difficult.

The difference in Carol's and Ron's activity levels can be seen in their daily routines. They maintain different schedules. Ron wakes up slowly and takes a lengthy hot bath. Carol has a special morning time for yoga and meditation. She commented, "Having my own house gives me the psychic and physical space to take care of myself."

They eat breakfast separately, each in his or her own home, often outdoors if the weather is fine. After breakfast, Ron goes to Carol's house for his morning hugs and kisses and for a discussion of their plans for the day.

"If I don't see Ron by 10 in the morning I begin to worry," said Carol.

Then during the day, each is busy with his or her own activities. Keeping up two houses and gardens is a lot of work. Carol takes classes, has recently earned her bachelor's degree, and is studying for a master's in alternative health care. Ron likes to shop, especially in hardware stores, and to have tea in his favorite café. Dinner together is by invitation. Carol has no television, but she and Ron sometimes watch TV together in his home, often with their arms and legs intertwined as they sit on his couch, hugging and kissing. Sometimes Carol spends the night with Ron, as he has the larger bed.

Ron is very romantic. Some years ago, when visiting a travel agent, he learned of a full-moon kayak trip. "It sounds very romantic," he told the agent. "I'd like to take my sweetie on one of those." And he did just that on Carol's birthday, under a full October moon.

Carol and Ron have a unique way of celebrating each other's birthdays. They start a month in advance, giving each other daily cards or gifts. "A gift could be doing the dishes for a week, or giving the other a massage or even a body lick. Any crazy thing," said Carol, laughing.

Sunday is a special time. They both dress up, go to church together, and often enjoy an elegant brunch afterwards.

Carol and Ron used to travel together a great deal. Now it is difficult for Ron to travel extensively. While they still take retreats together, Ron is mostly a homebody. Carol considers herself a "road warrior," taking off alone in her car, visiting friends, or just going to sit alone in the desert and meditate.

FINAL THOUGHTS

Despite conflicts and separations, Carol and Ron's love has held constant. Ron loves Carol unconditionally and shows it with daily affection. Carol recognizes Ron's basic trustworthiness and integrity. She states, "If a person has these qualities, other behaviors can be adjusted, and believe me, we've adjusted plenty." Their primary adjustment has been to live separately, and thus not be compelled to change habits and behaviors each considers essential.

Most important, they always have had the ability to nurture each other. Remember what sparked Carol and Ron's love? It was her covering him with a blanket that first cold, rainy night, and his bringing her coffee in the morning. They both recognized each other's needs and nurtured each other.

These caring qualities and loyalty remain. No matter what, Carol and Ron are there for each other. For them, the commitment of being married and the freedom of living separately is a successful **third option.**

Chapter 14

(Interview: Janice and Cliff)

THE LOVING IS EASY ... IT'S THE LIVING THAT'S HARD

With an expressive feeling, Cliff recites:

How can I tell you of my love?
Strong as an eagle.
Soft as a dove.
Patient as a pine tree that stands in the sun and whispers to the wind.
You are the one.

Janice glows as she listens. These words have important meaning for them both. Cliff saw the selection while on their honeymoon; he memorized it and had it framed. It is now on display in their house.

THEME
Developing Rules for Managing Conflict

Cliff and Janice have diametrically opposed styles of conflict. She's explosive, and he's uncomfortable with confrontation. From their deep commitment and love for each other comes their desire to adapt to each other's styles, and as a couple, they are developing their own rules for managing conflict.

INTRODUCING JANICE AND CLIFF

I was greeted by both Janice and Cliff, given a brief tour of their home, and ushered into the dining room where we held our joint interview. Janice, a recently retired child psychologist, is 55 years of age, of medium height and build, with lively brown eyes and a warm smile. Her short, curly hair is a salt and pepper color.

Cliff, age 67, a retired physical therapist, is tall and slender. He has gray hair, a gray beard, and warm brown eyes, with smile wrinkles around them.

They live in a house with a lovely view of rolling hills from the living area and master bedroom. The furniture is highly polished French provincial. A table in the living room is covered with framed photographs of Cliff's and Janice's families from early life through their marriage eight years ago. The house, owned by Janice, has been their home for five years.

HOW DID YOU MEET?

Janice had been single for 12 years after a divorce. She wanted to meet a man who was intelligent, educated, financially independent, and physically active.

> * It is good that Janice knew clearly the characteristics she wanted in a man as she began her search. We point out in Chapter 24 the need for this preparatory thinking before searching for a mate.

Janice had placed an advertisement in the personal column of the local newspaper, with no satisfactory results. Then one evening she had the opportunity to attend a singles-club dance, and there she met Cliff.

Cliff was also divorced and had been single six years. During that time he had been active in singles groups, and at meetings had listened to the viewpoints of other divorced persons. This helped him consider what he wanted in a woman.

> * Both singles groups and groups for the divorced can help a person look at what went wrong in a previous relationship and what traits might be desirable in a new partner. They also can help you explore what behaviors you can change as a new relationship develops.

That evening at the dance, Cliff stood at his customary spot by the wall until he asked a lady to dance. When the music stopped, he returned to the same location. Janice was standing there.

Cliff said, "You're standing at my place."

Janice replied, "I can stand here also. There's room for two."

They started a conversation and then danced together. As Janice exclaimed, "And it never stopped. We danced every dance together that evening. And then Cliff walked me to my car. I gave him my phone number and drove home. It took about 15 minutes to get home, and as I opened the door, the phone started to ring! That was the start, and we've been together ever since."

HOW WERE YOU ATTRACTED TO EACH OTHER?

Cliff answered this question by saying, "I immediately liked her conversational manner and wit. She sparkled, showing a lot of life. I was attracted to her looks, her face, and the way her hair was done. I really liked the care with which she put on her makeup, what she wears, and how she dresses in color-coordinated clothes. I appreciated her solid attitude about family and home. Janice is a different type of person than any woman I have known. She lets me know where she's coming from. She seems happy most of the time."

For Janice, these were features that attracted her to Cliff: "He was a good dancer and I liked that. I was also pleased with the neat way he was dressed and his athletic, trim figure. His conversation while dancing when we first met impressed me favorably. He talked about the sadness of children growing up in poverty. He pointed out the short sightedness of some social programs in not giving attention to after school care, nutrition, and family stability. These matters were important to me as a psychologist."

HOW DID YOUR RELATIONSHIP DEVELOP?

Their first meeting at the dance was just before Thanksgiving. Cliff then invited Janice to his home to join him and some of his friends for dessert on Thanksgiving day. She later asked him to accompany her to a friend's wedding reception. Thus, they started seeing each other through various activities in which each one was involved.

Janice continued, "I started to go to his house for dinner, and afterwards we would sit together by the fire. We loved to go dancing a couple of times a week. Our dating became very easy. We both saw our relationship from the first as something different and special. We certainly were attracted to each other."

A few weeks after Thanksgiving, Cliff helped Janice decorate her Christmas tree. She told him that she was planning to visit her family in Massachusetts. Cliff asked if he could go with her.

"That's pretty fast. I've known him less than a month," Janice thought to herself. She explained to me, "While single, I never had anyone visit my family at Christmas, but I did want to be with him and let my family meet him." She arranged the visit, and Cliff accompanied her. Thus, he was able to meet all of her relatives. It went very well.

"We were very smart," observed Janice. "We didn't jump into bed immediately. We did kiss and neck. Actually, we slept together a couple of times in each other's houses—*without sex*. It was three weeks before we had sexual intercourse."

> * Some couples interviewed would think that three weeks is a short time. Others had sex the night they met. The length of time a couple waits before having sexual relations, including those who wait until after marriage, depends upon their own value system.

Janice continued, "Since we both had been sexually active in recent months, each of us had a blood test that showed no presence of communicable diseases, including AIDS. As a further precaution, Cliff used a condom when our sex started."

> * Here they both were smart. There is evidence that older adults can and do contract AIDS. A blood test before sexual activity is a wise precaution.

Ten months after meeting, Cliff gave up his apartment and moved into Janice's house. To Cliff, "it felt like a ready-made arrangement—like home. Her elegant furniture and its arrangement in the rooms pleased me. We felt comfortable and stable together."

Janice agreed, "From the beginning, our relationship was not just trying it out. It was real."

> * There is evidence that couples who live together before marriage do not necessarily have a more stable marriage than those who do not. Wallerstein, in her book, *The Good Marriage*, writes about young couples who "play" at living together. (J. S. Wallerstein and S. Blakeslee,

> *The Good Marriage* (1995), New York: Warner Books, Chapter 14.)
>
> If, like Janice and Cliff, an older couple lives together with a determination to work out their differences and have a lasting relationship, the chances for a stable marriage are good.

Janice and Cliff lived together for a year and then decided to plan a traditional wedding. It took place at Janice's house, with 50 guests in attendance. These included both of their families and close friends. Following the ceremony, they took a cross-country honeymoon in their motor home. Shortly before the wedding, Cliff had retired, while Janice was still employed and needed to return to work. She flew back home, while Cliff, along with a brother, returned later in the motor home. This trip back across the country was leisurely, taking six weeks—a long time for newlyweds to be apart, but then they had been living together for a year.

When Janice and Cliff were asked, "Why was marriage important?" Cliff's reply was, "That's the way of telling the world I truly love the person I live with."

Janice followed with, "Marriage is a real commitment, and that's important to me."

Then two years after their marriage, Janice, who is financially more comfortable than Cliff, decided to purchase the house where they now live. Janice continued her lengthy commute to the clinic where she was employed. Since retiring, she has set up an office in the house to continue a small, private practice.

WHAT WERE YOUR EARLY LIVES LIKE?

Janice

Janice was raised in a working-class Italian family on the East Coast. She has only a younger brother. Her father was blustery, focusing on her faults. Her mother was high spirited, feisty, and argued easily. Despite the arguing, it was a close and loving family to whom Janice is very attached. Both parents are still alive, and she stays in contact, visiting with them and other family members as often as she can.

Cliff

Cliff grew up on a farm as the second youngest of 11 sons and 3 daughters. The whole family worked on the farm, and the children were a happy lot, although their upbringing was strict and church-going was enforced. He is still close to his brothers and his one living sister.

Janice and Cliff try to spend holiday times with both his and her families, usually alternating visits on both sides of the country.

WHAT WERE YOUR PREVIOUS RELATIONSHIPS LIKE?

Janice

At age 22, Janice started to live with a man who became her husband four years later. He was a salesman and developed an alcohol problem that, in time, became intolerable to Janice. They were together 12 years and then divorced. They had no children, which she always regretted. Her husband had a daughter from a previous marriage, who now has three children. Janice was close to the grandchildren during their upbringing and still is. She sees them three or four times a year and plans to provide for their education.

Following the divorce, Janice was single 12 years, during which time she completed her Ph.D. degree in psychology and became an employee in public clinics. Also, she was involved with a married man for eight years before meeting Cliff. Janice viewed that relationship at the time as "convenient, comfortable, and with few demands."

Cliff

Cliff was married at age 22 while in the service. He had two sons and now has six grandchildren. After the war, he became an insurance agent, but obtained a degree leading to a license as a physical therapist. He then was employed 25 years in that profession.

Cliff's marriage lasted 16 years, until irreconcilable differences arose. The differences became greater and they continued drifting apart until his wife initiated the divorce. She gained custody of their two children, which was very disturbing to Cliff. Now Cliff's sons and their six children all have good feelings for Janice, and she gets along well with them.

Cliff was single for six years, at which point he married again. In Cliff's words, "My new wife was brilliant but showed no common sense. She would insult people and not even realize it. I don't know why I married her. It was a mistake." This marriage lasted seven years. After that, Cliff had relationships that lasted from a few months to more than a year. He broke each one off, feeling it was not right for him.

As the result of his two divorces and his other involvements, Cliff became depressed. He received psychotherapy and attended a support group for the divorced. He also read extensively about developing good relationships and maintaining successful marriages. As he started to feel settled once again, he became socially active in singles groups. This eventually led to his meeting Janice. As Cliff thinks back, "Those women I knew were very different from Janice. She has a happiness and the ability to express positive emotions not found in my two previous marriages."

WHAT PROBLEMS WERE FACED AND WHAT ADJUSTMENTS WERE MADE?

Janice and Cliff recognize that they have different styles of conflict. Both agree that an individual's family background and upbringing can have important influences on behaviors in later life. Janice, being the first-born child, is well organized and doesn't rest until she has completed everything necessary. She believes she has a "critical parent" inside her and needs to control it.

On the other hand, Cliff, as the second youngest of 11 boys, has a laissez-faire attitude toward many things. Therefore, Janice says, "He has a natural exuberance and enjoyment for whatever he does. Wouldn't it be nice to be that carefree? I wish I could be more easy-going. Cliff tells me that he'd like to be more organized."

Cliff builds on this, "She's more serious about life than I am and takes more responsibilities."

* Here, as discussed in Chapter 18, good partners often have the same degree of emotional maturity but different character structures. Thus, they complement each other and help each other modify their more extreme behaviors.

Cliff and Janice's deep love for each other is a strong motivation for changing behaviors that cause the other pain. Janice expressed a "previous life" concept, saying, "I had a real sense we had been together before. We share similar life views and values, especially family values."

Despite this closeness, they do have difficulties. Following are some of their observations.

Remarks from Janice

"Small things bother me. He doesn't always close cabinet doors or put down the toilet seat cover. When I see such things not done right, my brain reacts and usually my mouth follows. I feel there's one right way to do things; therefore, I zero in on things not done properly. But I do appreciate things that he has done, like making breakfast for us. When I comment on his mistakes, it doesn't mean I don't appreciate the good things he's accomplished."

> * But does she openly express her appreciation? It is so easy to notice and comment upon a fault. We so often neglect to acknowledge what our partner has done right.

"Sometimes I'm just too uptight about small things that really don't matter so much. I look at him to help me loosen up. I am critical of his driving, which is maniacal at times. My reflexes are faster than his, so when I see something unsafe, I react quickly. He doesn't like that. We do argue back and forth at times and raise our voices—even call each other names. Frequently this happens when I'm tired, hungry, or cold. But these confrontations don't go on long. Sometimes he shouts, 'Stop it! Stop it! That's enough.' Shortly after the episode, we both say we are sorry about the disagreement."

> * Calling names can lead to deep hurts. It's good that Cliff shouts, "Stop it." It would be best if Cliff and Janice could separate earlier when angry and get back together when

calm. Janice could recognize when she is tired, hungry, or cold and thus, more likely to explode. Perhaps she could take care of herself in some way (meditation, a short nap, warm clothes, some food, or a hot drink) before taking up an issue with Cliff. After separating until calm, each could decide whether the issue is important enough to discuss at all.

As Janice says, "These periods of argument get me mad. Why do we have to argue? I'm beginning to realize that the things we argue about are not important enough to get upset over, and I'm gradually learning to hold my tongue."

Remarks from Cliff

"I know I'm not as organized as is Janice. She's more somber about life than I am. Also, she's super serious and responsible. These traits do cause some difficulties between us. We do have disagreements, and I feel vulnerable because I'm not used to having loud arguments. She's confrontational at times. Also, she talks emphatically with her hands at times. That's annoying. But I realize that her more spontaneous, outgoing style has helped me to recognize my emotional self. That is an important gift as you grow older. You can go one of two ways. You can be a bitter old man or a happy old man, and I am more and more a happy old man."

* Cliff's and Janice's ways of dealing with conflict might be attributed to their upbringing. Janice's family was Italian, and all members were very outspoken and loud. Arguing and shouting were normal behaviors for them. Therefore, she was used to that mode of behavior. Cliff's brothers and sisters learned early not to be confrontational; thus,

without such experiences, he was uncomfortable in face-to-face disputes.

Recognition of differences is a first step in modifying behavior. Janice is beginning to be less disturbed by Cliff's habits and is becoming more restrained in her reactions. Cliff is slowly learning to be more assertive and to both receive and express anger.

WHAT ARE YOUR ONGOING LIVES LIKE?

Janice observed, "Cliff and I have lives outside of our relationship. I love having time by myself, and he does also. To put it another way, we both have outside interests and lots to do. It is not always that I must be with him or he must be with me. When he is not here, I do more reading, watch old movies on television, do some correspondence, or edit a professional newsletter on the computer. He has become active in many community organizations in this area. He also spends a lot of time in our garden. Then, when we are together, it's even more special."

Janice and Cliff used to travel a good deal together, particularly to conferences and consultations in connection with Janice's professional work. Now, since they both have physical difficulties that limit their ability to exercise and even walk very much, they travel less. They frequently go out to dinner and spend evenings playing cards and watching television. Janice prefers light entertainment, while Cliff goes for historical programs. Because they have two receivers in the house, they sometimes watch separate programs concurrently. Sometimes they rent a video to enjoy old-time movies together, especially on a weekend when they can watch it in bed while eating dinner.

Cliff likes to read novels and nonfiction history, while Janice still reads her professional literature in addition to popular fiction and nonfiction.

Until a few months ago, Janice had a cat as a house pet, but it has died. Now they are preparing to acquire a dog for companionship.

* Pets can be an integral part of an older couple's family, almost like a new child. As a couple, you can share responsibilities for your pet, receive affection, and with dogs, walking them gives desirable daily exercise.

FINAL THOUGHTS

Some conflict is inevitable in any relationship. Cliff realizes this when he says "Marriage is made in heaven—so are thunder and lightning. We must live with it all."

Many couples come from different family backgrounds with different styles of conflict. This often is an advantage. If both partners are explosive, pandemonium can result. If both are very controlled, disagreements may never be dealt with, leading to growing resentment and disengagement.

Whether styles are similar or different, each couple needs to form their own explicit or implicit rules for managing conflict. Then each partner needs to modify his or her own behavior in accordance with these rules.

It isn't easy to be in an intimate relationship with another human being. It takes the love and commitment that Cliff and Janice so amply possess and the realization that, as so aptly expressed by Cliff, "**The loving is easy ... it's the living that's hard**."

Chapter 15

(Interview Barbara and Leonard)

AN IDEAL OLDER RELATIONSHIP—*IT'S A SMOOTHIE!*

"When I first met him, Leonard was good looking—WOW!—and he still is! We felt a lot of chemistry between us, but we knew it was not going anywhere."

"I've been a flirter all my life, and Barbara responded in the same way. I certainly wasn't straying from my loyalty to my wife, but this was casual fun between us."

That was more than 20 years ago. Now they are a happily married couple with an ideal relationship.

THEME
A Connection that Transcends Time

Have you ever had a special friendship with a person of the opposite sex where you knew on some deep level that here was someone you could trust and love? Barbara and Leonard formed such a friendship through their profession, and at the time, it was combined with a sexual attraction they were not free to act upon. After many years of no contact and then a lucky, brief meeting, Leonard communicated with Barbara, and they reestablished their relationship.

This reconnection occurs fairly frequently among older adults. Perhaps if you are single and longing for a partner, you could peruse your memories and locate a person with whom you had a bond in times gone by. Now that years have past, there is a chance that divorce or death of a spouse sadly may have made that person available again. And, if you reach out, you might also find that you and your friend have a connection that transcends time, as do Leonard and Barbara.

INTRODUCING BARBARA AND LEONARD

It took me some searching to find Barbara and Leonard's rural home, and I arrived a bit late for our interview. Both greeted me warmly and ushered me into a home that had been designed and charmingly decorated by Barbara.

Barbara is 64 years old, and Leonard is 70. They are both retired probation officers and at the time of our interview, had been married for one year. Barbara is a tiny woman, with short, straight gray hair and smiling hazel eyes. Leonard is more than six feet tall, slim, and balding. He is a handsome man with a square face and blue eyes. Both had a confident manner and were frank and open as we talked. Much affection was expressed between them—looking into each other's eyes, blushing while talking, and frequently touching each other.

HOW DID YOU MEET?

Barbara and Leonard served in probation departments in the same county but in different divisions: he in adult, she in juvenile. During their fairly frequent social gatherings, they became acquainted, chatting and dancing together, and sharing job experiences.

At that time, more than 20 years ago, Barbara was engaged and Leonard was married. But, as Barbara confided, "We felt a lot of chemistry between us, but we knew it was not going anywhere."

HOW WERE YOU ATTRACTED TO EACH OTHER?

These are some of Barbara's answers to this question:

"When I first met him, Leonard was so good looking—WOW!—and he still is! You can meet someone, and shortly thereafter you feel like you've known the person forever. There was that kind of rapport between us right from the beginning. We talked easily together—in the same language—probably because we were in the same occupation. And our thoughts flowed together so smoothly."

Leonard's observations about Barbara included these comments: "I liked her smile. It was a warm way of communicating and relating to me. She had a well-built body and she danced well. Her attitude about her work was very positive, and I admired that. I've been a 'flirter' all my life, and Barbara responded in the same way. I certainly wasn't straying from my loyalty to my wife, but this was casual fun between us."

HOW DID YOUR RELATIONSHIP DEVELOP?

After a number of years, Leonard transferred to another county. It wasn't until 15 years later that they encountered each other again under a different circumstance. Leonard had gone to an RV dealer for repairs on his vehicle. Barbara was there because she was getting ready to retire and was thinking about buying a small RV for traveling. They recognized each other, had coffee together, and visited.

By now, Barbara was divorced and Leonard, who had retired a few years previously, told her that his wife was ill with cancer. Because Barbara had suffered from breast cancer, she understood what Leonard was going through and sympathized with him.

A few years later, Leonard's wife died. Even though it was some years since he had last been in contact with Barbara, he wanted to talk with her, recalling that she, like his wife, had been through cancer operation and treatment. "She'll understand," he thought. Now, four months after his wife's death, Leonard found her phone number and called Barbara. She invited him to her house for lunch.

* As the result of a long-term study of happily married couples, Robert Levenson states, "I would argue that knowing how a person reacts when a partner expresses sadness is the most valuable piece of information to have if you're concerned about having a happy and lasting relationship." (*East Bay EXPRESS* newspaper, Berkeley, CA, July 9, 1999, page 9.)

Although Levenson doesn't use the words *compassion* and *understanding,* I believe that those are the reactions that need to be displayed when a partner expresses sadness. Barbara was able to do this, and Leonard was perceptive enough to recognize her ability to empathize with his pain. He sensed that she would be there for him as he grieved for his wife. This empathy between them was part of their original connection, and Leonard, in actively seeking out Barbara, reestablished their tie.

When Leonard arrived at her door, Barbara recalled, "He looked like a whipped puppy. Obviously he was miserable to have lost his wife to cancer after their 49 years of marriage." This was in early December, and it was apparent that there were still "sparks" between them.

During that visit, they made a New Year's date. Shortly thereafter, Leonard realized that January first was "too far away." He called, and they both decided to meet sooner. As they both agreed, "Things between us heated up fast." Leonard drove the 50 miles to Barbara's rural house, where they now reside. After three visits, he said to Barbara, "It's a long ride home for me. Can I stay overnight?"

"Sure," Barbara replied.

"Where can I sleep?" was the next question.

"Wherever you want to," came the response.

"That was it!" they both nodded and laughed together.

Following this meeting, they soon settled into a visiting pattern of every week, at least overnight and sometimes for a two-day period. Soon this visiting did not seem to be enough for either of them. Barbara had been enjoying her single life after a divorce. She could go where she wanted to and do whatever she desired, but "I did want him around, and I wasn't prudish about sexual matters. It didn't take long for me to hate it when he drove out of my driveway after a visit."

During his earlier married years, Leonard had felt that if anything should happen to take his wife, he would prefer to live with a woman but not get married. Now, Leonard stated, "When the time actually came, this idea didn't seem right." While both wanted to be together, it did not feel proper to live together unmarried. This could give the wrong impression to families and friends, especially so soon after the death of Leonard's wife.

* It is true that people can be shocked when a couple forms a new relationship soon after the death of a spouse. What they fail to understand is that a great deal of grieving and

of saying goodbye is often done during a long illness, and Leonard had nursed his wife for five-and-a-half years.

About a month after their New Year's date, they were engaged. When Leonard had first visited Barbara, he fell in love with her house and its land in the hills. They made the decision to live there.

Now that Barbara and Leonard look back at those times, they realize that Leonard never proposed marriage. They just understood it was what they both most wanted in order to bring them completely together. A simple, non-denominational wedding took place in May in the garden of Barbara's house. Leonard's son was the best man and Barbara's daughter was maid of honor. Family and close friends attended. Then Leonard moved a few of his possessions into Barbara's house, giving most of his furnishings to his children and disposing of the rest by having a garage sale. Together, they bought a king-size bed. Leonard is very comfortable in the house.

*   Parting with furniture may be difficult because it can symbolize giving up some of your past life with your spouse and the family you both raised. When children receive some of your possessions, you bequeath to them recollections of that earlier time, and your furniture is there for you to reignite these memories when you visit. Older individuals, especially, need a feeling of continuity, and memories are part of a complete sense of self.

    My city home holds 35 years of my earlier life. Now my daughter is living there with some of her furniture and some of mine, so that when I visit, I'm touching base with that long and significant time. Acknowledging and treasuring my previous life does not take away from the closeness that Jerry and I have now.

WHAT WERE YOUR PREVIOUS RELATIONSHIPS LIKE?

Barbara

Barbara was married for the first time at age 20, allowing her to get away from home. This marriage lasted for five years, during which time she had two girls. She supported her husband, who did not work regularly. He became physically and verbally abusive, and she divorced him.

One-and-a-half years later, she married a man 22 years older than she was. This marriage, while amicable, was not satisfactory, as they were far apart in their likes and dislikes. As Barbara said, "Our differences quickly caught up with us, and we parted after four years."

Barbara was then single for seven years. At age 38 she married again. This husband served as a father figure for her two girls, but he was a drinker and became assaultive. During this time, she developed cancer. Barbara commented on her situation during that period with this husband: "He was good to me during my illness, but as I recovered, my attitude toward myself changed. I became more aware of my own health, recognizing the need to take care of myself. He didn't understand me then. He frequently partied with his drinking buddies and didn't really care about me."

Barbara then insightfully expressed herself, "When someone contracts a cancer, he or she had better recognize what's important in life. I'd been completely a slave to my family. Now I realized I had to take care of myself and became more assertive in terms of my own needs. I had no consideration from my husband, so I started letting him know I was angry. I've learned that it's harmful to my body to internalize anger. I then decided I was going to beat this cancer. I gave my husband an ultimatum – either quit drinking or give me a legal separation." He left, and after 10 years, they divorced.

* There is a theory that internalized anger and a "too-nice personality" can lead to the development of cancer. Certainly, even if this theory is true, there are also other causes, such as hereditary and environmental factors.

When my late husband contracted prostate cancer, he went to a clinic that emphasized cognitive change. My husband learned to assert himself and pay better attention to his own needs. Possibly as a result, he lived longer than expected.

In Barbara's case, knowing that she had to take care of herself led to leaving a marriage in which her needs were not considered. This radical change in her life's outlook, I believe, led to her choosing Leonard—someone who fulfills her needs and brings her happiness.

When I asked Barbara to compare Leonard with her previous husbands, she made this observation: "There is no comparison. He's the gentlest man I've ever met. He's loving, sentimental, and so good. He's like a big teddy bear."

Leonard

At age 20, Leonard wedded his 18-year-old high school sweetheart. It was a good marriage that lasted 49 years, with two children, a boy and a girl. From the time when the first symptoms of his wife's cancer were detected, she lived five-and-a-half more years. Leonard took care of her until the end.

As Leonard described his feelings, "A year ago I couldn't have talked about her without crying. It still gets me a little bit. I turned to Barbara for comfort, and she has helped me greatly."

* I noted that as he talked, Barbara put her arms around Leonard and stroked his back. She continues to have the ability to empathize with his sadness, showing no jealousy of his former wife. This is an important part of their strong connection.

In addition to Barbara's comforting presence, living in her home has given Leonard a fresh start and has helped him recover from his grief. Both his wife and his mother died in the house where he had lived for many years, and it held many sad memories for him.

* It is interesting to note that leaving a family home is difficult for some but is a relief for others. Such a home may hold many precious memories of raising a family, and also memories of the illness and death of a loved one. **Ed,** as well as Leonard, found his family home filled with sad memories, and he was glad to leave.

WHAT ARE YOUR ONGOING ACTIVITIES AND INTERESTS LIKE?

In their marriage, Leonard and Barbara's closeness continues by sharing many pleasurable activities. Barbara receives much enjoyment from flower gardening, especially in growing roses, which were in full and fragrant bloom during my visit. Leonard likes to help with her gardening. She and Leonard spend quiet evenings reading. They seldom watch television. Leonard likes to tinker and is involved in many small construction projects. Every morning and evening they walk together on their property.

They both participate in various community services. Before meeting Barbara, Leonard had traveled little outside of his job requirements. Barbara, on the other hand, had taken many trips. Now they are traveling together, including their first ocean cruise to Hawaii.

Together they are taking a seminar about writing memoirs. Barbara encouraged Leonard to do this. He was somewhat reluctant at first, as he is not sure of his writing skills, but he is now enjoying the class.

> * Memoirs are an excellent way of finding a sense of continuity in life and sharing this life with children, grandchildren, and perhaps great grandchildren. **Nancy** and **Pat** also wrote their memoirs. When a couple writes the history of their lives together, they are sharing their personal stories with each other. This cannot help but add to a sense of closeness between them.

Barbara and Leonard spoke little of conflict in their marriage. Their adjustments in this area are covered in Chapter 18, *Personality Differences and Styles of Conflict.*

FINAL OBSERVATIONS

What is the basis of the strong connection between Leonard and Barbara? When they first knew each other, more than 20 years ago, they formed a genuine friendship, based partially on their common experience as probation officers. This mutual understanding of each other's past experiences enriches their present happy marriage.

When Leonard and Barbara first met, they felt a strong sexual charge between them. Because she was engaged and he was married, they had enough loyalty to their respective partners not to act upon this attraction. This restraint cannot help but have increased their respect for each other. Respect and an awareness of each other's basic integrity in both their professional and private lives were instrumental in their reconnecting more than 20 years later.

Because Leonard and Barbara had been good friends in years gone by, Leonard knew that Barbara was compassionate enough to help him with his grief. It might have been luck when they met again at an RV dealer's showroom, but Leonard deliberately sought Barbara out when his wife was dying. She continued to be supportive of him during his grieving.

Acceptance of a partner's sadness is a very important element in all relationships. Friendship, sexual attraction, basic integrity, and compassion are all factors in this connection that have transcended time and have led to an ideal older relationship.

Section Two

IMPORTANT TOPICS FOR OLDER COUPLES

Throughout their interviews, the couples replied to Edith's questions with information and descriptions of experiences covering a number of topics. In this Section, six significant topics are correlated and summarized. For easy reader reference, the names of the individuals and couples appear initially in **boldface** type. The pronoun *I* or reference to *Jerry and me*, are Edith's observations and reflections.

Chapter 16

RELATIONS WITH ADULT CHILDREN AND GRANDCHILDREN

Interactions with adult children are a very important aspect of almost every new, older couple's relationship. A study by the Gerontological Society of America gives evidence that a close, affectionate tie between adult children and their parents (or a parent) can contribute significantly to prolonging the parents' life. Most of our interviewees found acceptance from their children of their new relationship, but some, unfortunately, did not.

Adult children might have difficulty accepting their parent's new partner for various reasons. They may be very attached to the deceased parent and think it is disloyal for their mother or father to find a new love. They might be unwilling to share their parents' love or attention with another. Or, they might fear that they will lose part of their inheritance.

Often adult children have difficulty conceiving of their parents as sexual beings. It is not too different from young children who, when they learn the facts of life, find it hard to believe that their parents actually "do it." When I was a child, my grandmother remarried at a late age. My parents were glad that she had found a companion, but it was clear that they did not believe she could be sexual.

When Jerry and I got together, my daughter knew we were sexually involved but definitely did not want to know any details. "After all, you are my mother," she said emphatically. Certain boundaries need to be kept between parent and child. My daughter accepts Jerry.

She is an adult, so in no way is he a step-parent to her. She treasures her father's memory and enjoys Jerry's friendship and company. She is pleased that he makes me so happy.

Here are some examples from the couples interviewed, of both positive and negative interactions with children and grandchildren.

RUTH AND PAUL

Paul's wife, although still alive when he first became involved with Ruth, was suffering from Alzheimer's disease, and was completely incapacitated and uncommunicative. To marry Ruth, he had to divorce his first wife, while continuing to provide financial support for her as long as she lived. Paul talked with each of his three children, pointing out the many years he still had before him, expressing his desire to be free to have a better life with another woman. His children fully supported him. Ruth also wrote to Paul's children, telling them, "In no way would I take your mother's place. We'll just be companions to each other for the rest of our lives."

All their children, Paul's three and Ruth's daughter, attended their wedding and have happily accepted their new relationship. It is good that both Ruth and Paul communicated with Paul's children in advance, gaining their acceptance of his divorcing their mother to marry Ruth. Of course, they themselves were aware of their mother's decline with the disease, their father's care for her, and his lonely life when she became fully incapacitated.

KARIN AND JOHN

Karin resides separately from her partner, John. She has two sons, one of whom lives at a distance. He and his wife have met John briefly and have accepted his relationship with Karin. Another son and his wife live nearby. They have two girls. Karin baby-sits for them regularly. John has spent several nights at their home when Karin was baby-sitting, and the grandchildren have visited in Karin's house. The grandchildren are very fond of John. Recently, the three-year-old said, "I love ma-ma (grandma), and I love John too." When the grandchildren visit in Karin's home, they ask, "Where's John?"

John's four children have all met Karin and like her. John still spends holidays and birthdays with his ex-wife and adult children. This gives the children a connection with their past. Surprisingly, Karin accepts this situation with equanimity. Perhaps her living separately from John makes this easier for her. She might feel differently should they, in the future, live together or marry.

JOANNE AND ANDY

Joanne and Andy have a similar situation. They are not married but are living together. Andy's daughter resides nearby with her mother and visits often. She very much likes and admires Joanne, who had been helping her prepare for job interviews. However, her mother did not invite Joanne to the daughter's college graduation. This made Joanne extremely angry and hurt, though she realized that her lack of status as a "wife" and the relative newness of her relationship with Andy, were contributing factors.

One of two things would need to occur to change this situation that was so hurtful to Joanne. She could gradually come to accept not being included in his daughter's celebrations, or Andy could actively confront his former wife on Joanne's behalf, even to the point of refusing to attend an occasion himself unless Joanne was included.

Although their situations were similar, Karin and Joanne's reactions were different. I can only surmise the reasons for this difference. For one, Joanne lives with Andy, while **Karin** and **John** reside separately. Also, Joanne has a much more volatile personality than does Karin. There is no right or wrong reaction for not being included in an occasion involving your partner's children. Situations will differ, and the uniqueness of each individual needs to be recognized when attempting to resolve such a problem.

BARBARA AND LEONARD

Leonard, who is married to Barbara, has a son and a daughter, along with eight grandchildren. Barbara has two daughters and two grandchildren. Both had discussed the plans for their marriage with children and grandchildren. One of Barbara's daughters, and all of Leonard's family, accepted this event with pleasure. While Barbara is close to her one nearby daughter, it's Leonard's children and grandchildren who primarily make up their family.

When Leonard was first courting Barbara, his teenage granddaughter often took care of his dogs. After a few times, she became curious, asking him, "Where are you going grandpa? Are you seeing someone?" He answered by asking, "What would you say if I said, 'yes I am'?" His granddaughter replied, "I'd think it was wonderful."

As Leonard's son told Barbara, "You are really a mother to us all." And a grandchild, shortly before their wedding, asked Barbara, "Is it too soon to call you grandma?"

Leonard and Barbara actively communicated with their respective families as their relationship developed. Doing this can greatly ease the way for children and grandchildren to accept a new marriage or partners living together. It is unwise to surprise your children with a final decision.

NAOMI AND DAVID

With David and Naomi, both sets of children have had difficulty accepting the remarriage of their parents. At the beginning,

Naomi's daughters found it hard to accept David, as they had been very attached to their father. David's children had even more problems with the marriage than did Naomi's. One daughter used to call David daily, even after he married Naomi, but now that she, herself, is in a committed relationship, her constant need for her father has subsided. Naomi and David are agreeable to her present relationship and visit her and her partner every few months. The visits are cordial, but David tells me that both daughters, when on the phone, still speak to him disparagingly of Naomi, calling her an "old bitch." When they talk that way, he tells them to "go to hell."

It is sad that a situation like this cannot be resolved. It is good however, that David stands up for Naomi when his daughters speak negatively of her. If he didn't support Naomi, their marriage would surely suffer.

LAURA AND ED

Ed, age 90, has two sons, five grandchildren, and nine great-grandchildren. His wife, Laura, age 80, has a son and a daughter, a grandson, and two great-grandchildren. From the first, Ed was 100 percent accepted by Laura's family, and they have been very generous in paying for Laura and Ed's vacation trips. On the other hand, one son of Ed's and his family at first resented Laura, feeling that "no one could take mother's and grandmother's places."

Despite this resentment, Laura and Ed persisted in arranging pleasant, social contacts with Ed's family. They phoned, wrote often, and arranged gatherings at their home. Gradually Ed's children came to know Laura and to accept her as their father's new wife but of course, not replacing their mother in their hearts. Laura and Ed's persistence can be encouraging to those older couples who first do not find acceptance from adult children. They need to understand their children's attachment to a deceased parent and that forming a new bond takes time.

NANCY AND PAT

Nancy and Pat are a committed couple who are living separately. Nancy has two daughters, a son, and five grandchildren. Pat has seven children and 13 grandchildren. Nancy is closer to Pat's children than he is to hers. "Mother is all settled. Mother has her own life," says Nancy, referring to herself while waving her hands expressively. "Pat's children worried about someone taking care of him after their mother's death, and they see me as the caretaker for their daddy."

Often if a parent does not remarry or find a new companion, the children do become the sole caretakers when he or she declines. Adult children who are uneasy about a parent's becoming romantically involved should keep this eventuality in mind.

Nancy often visits her children alone. Pat takes her with him to see his children, and they all take trips together. Nancy showed me a photo of herself with her family. Pat was present when it was taken, but it was a family photo, and no one asked him to join in the picture-taking. "He really isn't part of my family, exactly," explained Nancy. But Nancy was planning to go with Pat to his granddaughter's wedding, and Pat said with directness, "I want you in the picture."

Nancy's children have all accepted her relationship with Pat, except for one daughter, who often expressed resentment. When Nancy sold her family home so she could buy the apartment in the retirement community near Pat's apartment, this daughter and her husband were extremely angry and hurt. In the past, Nancy had told her that she would eventually inherit the family home. Now she regrets very much ever saying this. Her advice to others is, "Never promise your home to any of your children. You never know what the future holds." I agree with Nancy's warning.

DONNA AND STUART

Stuart and Donna are a married couple with a 26-year age difference between them. He is 90 and she is 64. Donna has no children. Stuart's two sons accept Donna, but his daughter has been resentful toward her father's second marriage and has not been friendly to Donna. Donna believes that the daughter thinks she could not replace her mother in her life. Also, the fact that Donna is three years younger than the daughter, and is of a different religious denomination, are important factors affecting their relationship. Donna and this daughter planned a party for Stuart's ninetieth birthday, and although the party was successful, there was much dissension between them.

It is difficult for adult children to accept a parent's marrying someone who is close to their own age. I hope parents listen to and recognize their children's uncomfortable feelings, discuss their differences, yet hold firm in their allegiance to their spouses.

ELLEN AND RALPH

Ellen and Ralph are recently married. Of Ellen's three children, the two who live nearby have met Ralph and like him. But Ralph's four children, with whom he now does not have a strong relationship, have not clearly acknowledged his marriage to Ellen. His oldest daughter told him, "It was a stupid mistake for you to marry." Ralph has tried to convince his children to change their attitudes, expressing hope that "Once the die is cast, let's accept the results." From Ellen's position, it is understandable when she says, "I do not feel welcome in his family."

After their mother's death, when these adult children were young, Ralph had married a woman 16 years younger than himself. His new wife disliked the children, and they hated her. This unhappy experience might be affecting their attitude toward Ellen.

GAYLE AND JIM

Gayle and Jim are living together and plan to marry shortly. Gayle, a widow, has a daughter with one child and an unmarried daughter. Although Gayle and her daughters are very close, her unmarried daughter has not established rapport with Jim, even though he is a very warm and open person who is easy to know and to like. Perhaps her reserve is because Jim is 10 years younger than Gayle, or because she was close to her deceased father. Or, Gayle's daughter possibly does not want to share her mother's love and attention.

Jim has a young adult son from his marriage and is now completely alienated from him; there is no contact. Jim attributes this to the influence of his former wife. Also, before he met Gayle, he and his former wife were considering re-uniting. His union with Gayle must have been a shock and a disappointment to his son. I find that children, no matter what age, hope their divorced parents will eventually be reunited. This brings up the subject of alienation from adult children.

ALIENATION FROM A CHILD

Fifteen couples are described in this book. Of these 30 individuals, 3 were completely alienated from one or more of their children, having no contact with them at all. I believe this 10 percent is a reasonable number but unfortunately, a high one.

Seymour has three daughters. The oldest and the youngest chose to feud with the middle daughter, while Seymour supports this middle daughter. As a result, he has no contact with two daughters, and it is only the middle one with whom he and **Edna** have a relationship.

Barbara and **Leonard** enjoy close contact with Leonard's two children and one of Barbara's daughters. But Barbara is completely alienated from her other daughter, having no contact with her. She gave no explanation for this rift. Perhaps she doesn't understand it herself.

Losing contact with an adult child is not only painful but also is socially embarrassing. It doesn't fit the picture of many generations of a happy family, all loving each other and getting along well. Also, others might think the alienation must, in some way, be the parent's fault. It is my opinion that most people do not freely share with others this loss of contact with an adult child. We certainly don't read about it in Christmas letters! Alienation from an adult child probably is much more common than most of us realize.

Though **Jim**, **Seymour**, and **Barbara** must feel pain from losing their children, they have not let the sadness interfere with their present happy lives. The same can be said for all those individuals whose children have difficulty with their new relationships. Those who have happy, successful partnerships, or those working toward greater compatibility, recognize that their new relationship is vital to them at this time of their lives. It is wonderful when all the children are close and there is full acceptance of the new relationship. Family is so important, and large, happy family gatherings, sometimes involving several generations, can be memorable. But we know this is not a perfect world, and mature adults have learned to accept what *is* and treasure the love they have for each other.

IN SUMMATION

Our couples have experienced both positive and negative interactions with their children and grandchildren. Whatever your situation, loyalty to your new relationship should be primary. I recently counseled a man who was distraught because his new wife had left him. It was his involvement with his adult children's many problems that had greatly stressed his marriage.

Good relations with each other's families need to be encouraged early. This can be done by honestly communicating with your children as the new relationship develops and by arranging pleasant activities together. Do not surprise your children and grandchildren by suddenly announcing your upcoming marriage to someone new to them. Let them know they are still important in your life and that you do not expect your new partner to replace their parent in their hearts. Also, inform your children that you have not forgotten them in your will. (See the section about wills and trusts in Chapter 26 for advice about how to provide for your children.) Your children also need to know that, should your health fail, your new partner may be able to help with your care. These communications can smooth the relations between children and your new partner, making for happier family interactions.

Chapter 17

HEALTH AND SEXUALITY

One of the most inspiring lessons I have learned from the couples interviewed is that physical intimacy is an important and satisfying part of their relationship. And of course, health, especially in later years, is inextricably tied to sexuality.

A study of the sex life of older Americans, age 60 or older, that was conducted in 1998, shows that many older persons are active sexually. The following was reported:

- 71% of men and 51% of women in their 60s were sexually active, while 57% of men and 30% of women in their 70s were sexually active. (These percentages might be low because, as well as recently coupled older people, the study included both single individuals and long-married couples.)

- When asked about the emotional satisfaction they receive from their sex life, 74% of sexually active men and 70% of active women said they were as satisfied or even more satisfied than they were in their 40s. (We had quite a few couples who said the same!)

- When older people are not sexually active, it is usually because they lack a partner or because they have a medical condition.

(Study conducted by *National Council on Aging*, Washington, D.C., as reported in their Web page: http://ncoa.org/archives/sexsurvey.htm)

The dark side of this sexual activity is that older adults are becoming increasingly vulnerable to infection with the HIV virus (see statistics on page 283). A blood test for AIDS is a wise precaution before becoming involved sexually.

Physical changes occur gradually as both men and women age. After menopause, women can suffer from vaginal atrophy, a thinning of the vaginal wall, that can result in pain during or after intercourse. Oral estrogen and estrogen cream applied to the vagina can often alleviate this problem. There is also a decrease in vaginal lubrication, especially if a woman is not taking a form of estrogen. Here, an over-the-counter lubricant applied before intercourse is very helpful.

Men gradually begin to have less firm and less frequent erections and more limited ejaculations. This will vary greatly with the man's health. While impotence often is assumed to be part of the normal aging process, this is not necessarily so. Rather, it may reflect the effect of such chronic diseases as diabetes. Arteriosclerosis and hypertension can affect the blood vessels and therefore, the firmness of erection. Often necessary medications can interfere with sexual function, especially those used to treat heart disease, high blood pressure, depression, and anxiety. But even with the changes of aging, the impact of diseases, and the effects of drugs, older couples can to some degree, continue to enjoy a satisfying sex life.

Not all serious medical conditions interfere with sexuality. Particularly inspiring were three women who had medical problems that one would think could end their chances of being sexually attractive to a partner. **Karin** had a mastectomy, losing one breast, and **Barbara** lost two breasts with a double mastectomy. **Naomi** had an ileostomy after suffering from colon cancer and must defecate into an external bag. All of these women had these operations before they met their present partners yet were able to be attractive to their mates and then to enjoy their sexual lives.

Sex is not just a physical act. It is a supremely bonding force between a loving couple. For Jerry and me, our sexuality has formed a strong tie between us, leading to much affection, teasing, and laughter. It makes our problems seem less important and adds immeasurably to the "we" between us. Both of us had seriously ill spouses and long periods of abstinence, so our lovemaking makes up for those years without it. If continued aging or medical problems catch up with us, we will still be sexual to some degree, and the bond will have been formed.

The couples we interviewed have taught us a great deal about sexuality in later life. For all of them, the return to a sexual life was an important part of their relationship. Here are their stories.

RUTH AND PAUL

Ruth, age 78, and Paul, 80, a married couple, are an inspiration. When they first became sexually involved, she was 71 and he was 73. Their first experience together, after many years of abstinence, was not satisfactory. In fact, Ruth said it was "terrible." She had a yeast infection and had suffered from vaginal dryness, which now is successfully treated with hormones.

Especially after long years of abstinence, it takes time for a couple to be sexually comfortable again. With time, trust, and good communication, a sexual rhythm can be found. As time passed, Ruth and Paul became more comfortable together, and their sex life gradually improved. Now they have sexual activity almost daily, after waking in the morning. (With most couples interviewed, morning is the prime time for sex, probably because they are rested.) When stimulated, Ruth attains orgasm and finds the experience "lovable."

They both believe that "sex contributes much to holding a marriage together. It increased the bond between the two of us. We express every day our love for each other."

At age 80 Paul has no problems with penal erection or ejaculation! This is somewhat unusual, but Paul is active, in good health, and looks to me like a man of 60. He has a slightly enlarged prostate gland that is controlled with medication, but that does not interfere with his enjoyable sex life.

NANCY AND PAT

Nancy, age 75 and Pat, 77, are a committed couple living separately. Let Pat tell us how their love life developed.

"The physical attraction to Nancy grew on me naturally. I just got to liking her better and better. I didn't have any idea at first we'd ever do anything sexual. Then one night as we were cuddling up watching television, I just happened to mention, 'I wonder if we could go to bed together.' Laughingly, we ran into the bedroom ... and so it started."

It was after the beginning of their sex life that Nancy and Pat started to spend nights at each other's homes and to see themselves as a committed couple. With most of those interviewed, their first sexual encounter also marked the beginning of their commitment to each other.

At present Nancy and Pat have intercourse about twice a week, usually in the morning. At almost age 77, Pat still is able to hold an erection but doesn't always ejaculate. "I can only charge up my battery twice a week," he said with a smile. Pat feels he is able to enjoy sex more with Nancy than he had with his wife, primarily because during their marriage, as Catholics, they used the rhythm method for contraception. "It didn't work very well—we had seven children. But maybe it did, since we didn't have 14!"

Nancy had a hysterectomy at age 45 and takes estrogen. She lubricates naturally and is orgasmic. She suffers from incontinence however, and has had surgery for this problem. She presently uses pads, but this in no ways turns Pat off sexually. Sex is better for her with Pat than it was with her husband, but at that time, between her husband's work and the raising of three children, their distractions from sexual intimacy were many. For her, as a Catholic, the rhythm method was an interference until after her hysterectomy. Also, her husband was more inhibited than is Pat. "I'm a much different person now with Pat. We have a very open relationship sexually. He is a great lover. We can talk freely about our love life. I'm very responsive."

JOANNE AND ANDY

Joanne, 59, and Andy, 60, are a younger couple than most of those interviewed. After dating 14 months, they have now been living together for eight months. They became sexually involved after keeping company for seven weeks. Joanne "held out" that long because Andy had told her that with his participation in singles groups, "The easiest thing in the world was to get laid." She didn't want to be "just another lay." At first, they necked and petted. "It was like being in high school, in the back seat of a car, steaming up the window," Joanne recalled. "The first time we had intercourse, it wasn't the best sex, but it's been getting better ever since."

Joanne has a stronger sex drive than does Andy. "I take hormones and would like sex almost everyday," she said. Andy had a previous bout with cancer, which somewhat lessened his energy level and thus, the frequency of his sexual desire. They have sex about once a week, and Joanne has learned to accept this. With a pleased look on her face, she exclaimed, "After living five years by myself, I thought I liked sleeping alone. Now I practically sleep on top of him, like a fly on a windshield." Andy, with a glow on his face, added, "Just feeling our bodies close. It's really nice. In the morning when we cuddle and hold each other, to me that's heaven."

Disproving earlier stereotypes, it is not at all uncommon for many women to want intercourse more frequently than do men. Closeness in bed, which Joanne and Andy so much enjoy, is a pleasure that can be savored for many years, despite increasing age and deteriorating health.

KARIN AND JOHN

Karin and John, like **Pat** and **Nancy**, are a committed couple, living separately. Their intimate relationship started about two years ago. Both are presently in good health, although in the past, Karin underwent a mastectomy, losing one breast. The loss of her breast did not stop John from finding her desirable, nor did it interfere with their sexual pleasure.

John, 69, tends to be a worrier. Thus, when discussing sexuality, he, in his introspective way, expressed concern about his sexual performance. I dislike that word *performance* when men use it. It detracts from spontaneity and seems to put pressure on the man "to perform." It seems that Karin, at 65, would like sex more frequently than would John. He realizes that often he is tired from too much activity such as running and dancing. John often reaches ejaculation before Karin climaxes and then satisfies her manually. She expressed the wish that they could climax together during intercourse. When I discussed this with the two of them, they both realized that this goal was based on a myth. It is seldom that both partners climax at the same time.

John was concerned that he no longer could achieve an erection by just thinking about Karin, as he did when he was younger. Men can do this in their teens and early twenties, but certainly not at age 69! His erection now takes longer to attain, but this is no problem if he takes time, relaxes, and caresses Karin. Also, his erection doesn't last as long as it did when he was younger. John needed reassurance that this is all normal as a man ages. When the three of us discussed their sexuality together, John made a wise statement to my explanation of normal erectile changes with aging. He responded with, "If a man doesn't know these facts, he can get scared and then may really not get it up."

Karin has none of John's worries. She described their sexual life as "wonderful, open, and satisfying." Although it had been many years since she had been sexually involved, she has had no problems with urinary tract infections or vaginal dryness. She has multiple orgasms, and John really likes that. Karin observed, "John has an amazing ability to turn me on." She sometimes would like sex when John is not in the mood but is accepting of this and hopes John doesn't feel pressured, which he doesn't.

It was delightful to talk with this couple together about their sexual relationship. They were very open, and their faces glowed. While talking, they would sometimes touch each other's hands or knees. When asked about sexual frequency, they agreed it was usually once or twice a week. The more they are together, the more frequently they are sexual if they are rested and not too busy. With a twinkle in his eye, John said, "If my friends read this, tell them we have sex at least three times a week!"

I laughed and said to John, "You worry too much." John responded, "I do." Karin smiled, saying, "He's a worry wart."

JANICE AND CLIFF

Janice, age 55, and Cliff, 67, are married and have been together as a couple for about eight years. For many years, their sexual intercourse was very satisfactory, but now the activity is "much quieter." Cliff had a diminished sex drive and difficulty maintaining an erection. In discussing sexuality with them, Cliff expressed the fear that he was impotent. Janice believed that she had lost her attractiveness to him, while he had refrained from approaching her because of his performance anxiety.

Janice said, "Sex is an important part of our relationship, and I miss it. We both feel insecure about Cliff's condition, knowing that otherwise he is in good health. As his desire reduces, he does worry about his performance."

Then in our discussion, Cliff was relieved to learn that to some degree, problems with erection are common with aging. This knowledge has decreased his anxiety so that now he maintains a firm erection and their sex life is improving. If a man does not understand these natural changes and believes he is impotent, this thought alone is enough to inhibit his erections. Cliff also saw his doctor and was prescribed Viagra™, which he uses on occasion. Since Cliff reports that his health is excellent, I believe it was his performance anxiety that caused the problem. Janice is pleased that sex is now more frequent and satisfying. "If I'm not getting enough sex, I'm somewhat edgy." The two do touch, snuggle, kiss, and at times, mutually masturbate.

NAOMI AND DAVID

David, age 80, has similar concerns about impotence. He and Naomi, age 78, a married couple, have been together 14 years. Naomi told me that when they first became sexually involved, they had an active and enjoyable sex life.

Now approaching 81, David admits sadly that he is impotent. The most likely cause is the medication he has been taking for high blood pressure. Recently the dose was lowered, and Naomi said, "If he's off the full dose now, we'll see what happens."

This impotence is of great concern to David. He tried a suction pump, but it hurt, and now wants to use Viagra™, but "Naomi won't let me." She's afraid it might harm him. When Naomi, David, and I discussed sexuality, Naomi emphasized that David brings her to orgasm by stimulating her clitoris with his hand, and I pointed out that for many women, clitoral stimulation may be even more satisfying than intercourse.

Naomi was emphatic about David's concern regarding his lack of erection: "It's no problem for me. It is only a problem for him. For him it's in his head. We have sex about once a month now. It's good enough for me. I'm not 21 years old. If only sex were what I wanted with David, would our relationship have lasted this long?"

CAROL AND RON

Carol, age 64, and Ron, 82, have been together 17 years. They are married and live separately. When they first became involved, at ages 47 and 65, they had many periods of intensive, unfettered sexual activity, although Carol reported that from the first, while she had satisfying orgasms, she also experienced discomfort. Then, because of a back problem and vaginal pain during intercourse, she lost her sex drive and now has no desire for sexual relations. "It hurts too much. I can't stand it." Carol attributes her vaginal pain and problems with sexuality to having been molested as a child. She recovered memories of this abuse as an adult, during individual and group therapy.

The theory behind "recovered memories" is that severe physical and sexual abuse is too painful for a child to hold in consciousness. These memories are therefore, dissociated (kept out of consciousness) and recovered in later years, usually during psychotherapy. There is much dispute in the psychotherapeutic community about the validity of this theory. My stance is that it is possible for a child to dissociate from painful experiences and recover them later, in or out of therapy. However, far too many therapists and support groups actively suggest and lead clients to what is now considered by some as "false memories." Considering that Carol was left alone and unprotected a great deal as a child, I believe that her memories are most likely true.

About five years ago, Ron was diagnosed with cancer of the prostate. He had an orchiectomy that removed the testosterone-forming glands from his testicles to retard the spread of the cancer. As a result, he lost his ability to have an erection. Carol and Ron no longer have sexual intercourse, and Ron finds this frustrating. Their feelings for each other are expressed by sitting together, holding hands, and hugging, but no strong kissing, touching, or stroking of intimate parts. They sleep together at times, in a companionable way. Carol told me that Ron sees intercourse as the only way of making love, and he is not willing to "do other things" that she would find exciting and satisfying.

SOME SUGGESTIONS

Older couples need to know that there are many other ways to achieve sexual arousal and even orgasm other than through intercourse, or in addition to intercourse. The following suggestions may be helpful if they fit with your religious convictions and sexual preferences.

Touching the breast and stimulating the nipple with the hand or tongue can be very exciting. There is a spot right at the bottom of the spine that is erogenous. In fact, tenderly stroking and kissing all parts of the body can be a loving and exciting experience for both the receiver and the giver.

Mutual masturbation with the man gently rubbing the vulva and clitoris with a moist finger, and the woman stroking the penis can often lead to orgasm. The penis, limp or erect, can be rubbed within the exterior vulva and against the clitoris. Then there is oral sex, a very common practice today. In cunnilingus, the man stimulates the woman's outer vagina and clitoris with his tongue. This can be extremely exciting and often the only, or the main way, that many women achieve orgasm. Fellatio refers to the woman sucking a man's penis. With this procedure, a woman can give her partner excitement and bring him to orgasm. She can withdraw her mouth before ejaculation, if desired. Two references treat this topic:

- *The New Male Sexuality,* by Bernie Zilbergeld, 1992; Bantam Books (particularly pages 108–111, and 357–358)

- *The New Joy of Sex,* edited by Alex Comfort, 1996; Crown Publishers (particularly pages 85–88 and 105–110)

SEXUAL BEHAVIORS OF OUR OLDEST COUPLES

Here is a brief look at some of the oldest couples in the book to see how their sex lives have changed over time.

Mary and **Fred** married when she was 63 and he was 57. Now she is 85 and he is 79. Previously they had an active sex life during their marriage. Now their sexuality is "nice," but they both agree that Fred's erectile capacity is affected because of his medication for heart problems and diabetes. Mary states that "sex is not everything in a marriage." Fred follows with, "You get satisfaction from kissing and holding hands, and also closely embracing each other while in bed."

Laura, age 80 and **Ed**, 90 relate that for both of them, sex at first was "very healthy," with intercourse three to four times a week.

Their relationship started at ages 60 and 70. But over time, with surgery and medications, Ed's erection has lost its firmness. At 90, Ed has had his share of severe medical problems, particularly with his heart and circulation system. Now hugs and kisses are more important for expressing their affection.

Stuart is 26 years older than **Donna**. When first married, both of them felt their sexual activity was "good" (two to three intercourses a week). Consider his age when they married—78! Now, at age 90, Stuart can experience only limited penal erection, and they try for intercourse about once a month. For his 90 years, Stuart is in good health. He has had no surgeries and takes no medication. However, with a general slowing down, certainly expected at his age, it is difficult for Stuart to move to various body positions during intercourse.

Donna often feels excited and misses sexual activity with Stuart, and she initiates some playfulness through physical touching. As Stuart says, "It's up to her now if she gets the desire." This discrepancy of desire is to be expected with Donna being so many years younger than Stuart. It is good that she is able to initiate some activity.

All three of these oldest couples had frequent intercourse when they married at a fairly late age. Now, because of medical conditions, their sex life consists primarily of affection and physical closeness. They have had enough years together to enjoy sexual intimacy and become more deeply bonded. The suggestions I offer for sexual practices, other than intercourse, would not fit for these oldest couples because of their possible conservative orientation, and it might not be necessary because they are content with their love lives as it is now.

IN SUMMATION

All the couples had active and satisfying sexual lives during the early parts of their relationships. For those who married, only those with strong moral and religious convictions against pre-marital sex waited until after marriage to become sexually involved. Some, like **Ruth** and **Paul,** have continued with frequent and enjoyable intercourse until very late in life. Other couples, because of physical problems and medications, no longer have intercourse but still enjoy much affection and cuddling in bed.

For many couples interviewed, their frequency of sexual activity lessened as they aged. A sense of humor can greatly help if this occurs. With a smile and a nod of his head, one interviewee told me this story about two men conversing in a barber shop:

"Do you remember the first time you had sex?"

"I can hardly remember the last time I had sex."

"That may be true for you, but I have sex *almost* every day … *almost* on Monday, *almost* on Tuesday, *almost* on Wednesday…."

For older individuals, it is important to know that certain changes in erectile functioning and ejaculation for the man, and thinning of the vaginal walls and a decrease in lubrication for the woman, are normal with the aging process. This can greatly relieve anxiety so that the couple may continue to enjoy a satisfactory sexual experience.

Chapter 18

PERSONALITY DIFFERENCES AND STYLES OF CONFLICTS

How often have you seen the very talkative, outgoing wife or husband with a quiet partner? What would a relationship be like if both partners were impulsive? Who would put a stop to unwise actions or decisions? What if both were subdued and restrained? Who would add spirit and excitement to the relationship?

For many years I have observed that good partners often have the same level of emotional maturity while being of opposite personality types. Thus, in their togetherness they complement each other.

If one partner is imaginative and spontaneous and the other more down to earth and practical, they can balance each other and add a great deal to each other's lives. One can bring new interests and excitement into a partnership; the other can offer safety and stability. The trick is to appreciate the differences and what your partner has to offer, rather than strive for a carbon copy of yourself. Conflict can result from personality differences, or these differences can be appreciated. Also, different personality types address conflict in different ways, from volatile outbursts to withdrawal.

This chapter addresses the similarities and differences in the personalities of our couples and the ways they approach conflict. Some conflict is inevitable in all relationships, and newly formed older couples, with their longstanding habits and opinions, certainly have plenty of areas for disagreements. At the end of the chapter, you will find *Dos* and *Don'ts* for handling conflict.

Understanding how your partner's personality differs from yours can help you not to become offended when you fail to get a particular reaction you are expecting. I found this very much so with my late husband. After I had purchased a new outfit, I often would approach him with, "How do you like this?" as I stood before him proudly modeling my new dress. I meant the big picture: "How do I look in this new dress?" and "What is your overall impression?" I would be very annoyed when he would look only at small details: "The hem is uneven." Or, "I like the embroidery on the collar."

Sometime into our marriage we both took a personality test—the *Myers-Briggs*—to learn more about ourselves. (This test is available online at http://www.humanmetrics.com/infomate/infoMatePass.asp) We discovered that I was highly *intuitive.* This meant that in a situation, I would consider the *big picture* by grasping essential patterns, as was fitting with my profession as a psychotherapist. My husband scored high on the *sensate* scales indicating that he used his eyes, ears, and other senses to find out what was actually happening around him. The results showed that he was practical, being good at working with facts and examining details. That could explain his engineering background and why his attention was directed at seeing only the details of my clothes. After learning that he perceived the world as a *sensate* individual, not seeing the big picture as I had wanted him to, I felt much less disturbed by his comments about my attire.

Jerry, like my late husband, is much more organized and practical than I am. He brings these abilities into our lives and also into this book. Conversely, I like to think that I've brought more richness and adventure into his life. Often I see or hear of a trip that appeals to me, and my first thought is, "Let's go!" Jerry is more hesitant, but if we do go, he enjoys himself immensely.

Though Jerry, like my late husband, is sensate and I am intuitive, we are both extroverted. In social situations and when speaking in public, each of us has trouble getting a word in edgewise while the other one is talking. This could make for conflict, but knowing each other's behavior in such situations, we find it amusing.

A few of the couples were very clear about how their personalities complemented each other. Some were explicit about how they handle conflict. Others claimed to have no differences, but areas of disagreement and how they were dealt with gradually came out during the interviews.

JOANNE AND ANDY

Joanne and Andy are particularly clear about how their differing personality traits are complementary. Joanne describes it as "the show girl and the intellectual." She likes rock music; he prefers classical. He likes artistic foreign films; she prefers American romance and adventure.

Joanne lives and works at a fast pace, which Andy admires but doesn't want to get dragged into. Andy is slower, more thoughtful, and introspective. She feels like "winding him up"; he feels like "slowing her down." But at the same time, Joanne agrees with many of Andy's efforts to ease her pace, as she tends to over-work and over-book herself.

Joanne prefers to live on a grander scale financially than does Andy. He says, "I shop in Target, she shops at Nordstroms." Joanne appreciates Andy's helping her to be more careful in her spending, as she has a tendency to go overboard. Andy appreciates Joanne's helping him to be more expressive. He finds it easier now than ever before to show love and tenderness.

Joanne has a temper and will yell and call Andy names when she is angry; however, she gets over it quickly and doesn't hold grudges. Andy is more self-contained and introspective. He doesn't show anger and tends to hold it inside, but Joanne senses his displeasure.

Both Joanne and Andy, as children, had problems with their fathers, but they respond differently to conflict. This is not unusual. Even children in the same family will develop different personality traits in dealing with the same parents. Joanne's father was volatile, and she in turn, learned to have a short fuse, thus her quick temper in arguments with Andy. Her marriage with her second husband, an explosive man like her father, did not work out at all.

Andy's father was a stern disciplinarian who frequently beat his sons. Andy protected himself as a child by walling himself off from being expressive. Thus, he tends not to show anger, but to hold it inside. He expresses anger in more subtle ways and admits, "I can be a bully like my father." Joanne doesn't let him get away with this bullying, and Andy says with admiration, "This woman can't be frightened."

NANCY AND PAT

Nancy and Pat had taken the *Meyers-Briggs* test. Nancy referred to the findings for explaining their personality differences. Nancy, like my late husband, is a sensate type; practical, organized, and settled. Pat is disorganized, perceptive, and thinks ahead. An intuitive-type like me, Pat is enthusiastically planning the next trip while they are still engaged in a present adventure. He has brought a good deal of excitement into Nancy's life and much openness and freedom to their sexual experiences. Nancy offers Pat stability and organization, which he gratefully accepts. For example, he gives her his bills to pay and accepts her reminders of appointments without resentment. In this good match, during their later years, each partner has found in the other undeveloped parts of themselves.

Both tell me that they never had an argument. This is hard to believe, but they assure me that it is true, and I don't see the distance between them that repression of conflict often brings about. They do say they have “heated discussions” at times. When I saw Nancy and Pat together, they gave me an example of such a discussion. When Pat sold his house, he gave the new owners his washing machine and dishwasher. Then he asked if he could leave his tent trailer in the garage for three days. They refused. Indignantly, he told Nancy, “They wouldn’t let me do it! After all I’ve given them.”

Then Nancy stated, “I was the voice of reason.” To Pat she said, “They paid you $14,000 extra for the house. They might have need for the space.”

Pat replied, “She’s more forgiving that I am. She’s nicer than I am. Anyone who pulls a dirty trick like that on me, I’m through with them.”

Nancy continued, “So I said, ‘We have to get out the phone book and call a towing service,’ and in no time, the trailer was up here.” At that point, they both laughed, and Pat concluded, “How did I know it was going to be so easy?”

This example points out the difference in their approaches. Pat was indignant and explosive in describing the situation. Without Nancy’s calming influence, he might have had quite a dispute with the buyers of his home. Nancy and Pat were both able to laugh about the situation. Humor is a great softener of disputes. In addition, the fact that this couple lives separately makes for less of the day-to-day frustrations that cause conflicts.

ELLEN AND RALPH

Ellen and Ralph had a good deal of conflict in the early “working out” period of their relationship. Their different personality styles were evident in their arguments. Ellen told me, “We have heated discussions, and I get very verbal. He pulls back and becomes defensive and quiet. He's analytical and thinks things through much more than I do."

To confirm this, Ralph later confided, " I approach things in a logical way. She's not logical; she's very emotional." To use the *Meyers-Briggs* dichotomy, Ellen is a "feeling" type, and Ralph is a "thinking " type. This difference was gradually understood by both of them so that neither felt offended by the other's style, and their relationship is much improved.

GAYLE AND JIM

In meeting Gayle and Jim, one factor soon became clear to me. Gayle is extremely energetic, talkative, and constantly on the go. Jim is much quieter. Gayle is aware of this difference and remarks, "Jim is more laid back that I am. The time factor between us is different. I believe in doing something right now. He thinks before acting. He slows me down. I accept the difference, and now I don't get as upset. I really don't think I would have been amenable to this sort of change at a younger age. As you get older, you become more realistic of what can be accomplished in life."

This is an encouraging comment. If older individuals are more realistic, it could balance the problem of having longstanding habits and attitudes later in life. In turn, Jim states, " I had been less organized than she. I let things go. I was messy. Now I get to important things quicker and am neater."

Like **Cliff**, Jim credits his partner with helping him to be more aware with his emotional side. "I realize that I have changed in my life with Gayle. I'm more in touch with my tender feelings. She has helped me work through some issues I had buried. Life has opened doors for me, giving me more choices to make than previously. These choices provide opportunities to grow that I had not had before meeting Gayle. I feel at home here with her."

"It's important to enjoy life," Gayle continued. "Savor and make good use of the time you have. I've learned from Jim how to play. We sit by the river and look around at our world together. That helps to make a good life for us."

I felt very moved by these comments. As with other couples interviewed, Gayle and Jim's differences benefited them. Jim has become neater, more organized, and punctual. Gayle has learned to slow down a little and to relish life. Through their relationship, each has become a more complete and happy person.

BARBARA AND LEONARD

This couple is an example of the "non-bossy" approach being very helpful. Barbara, like **Ellen**, worked in a setting where she was in charge and gave orders. She knew that she was somewhat "bossy," as she often had to give directions to probationers. When she feels under pressure with, for example housework, she has learned not to give an order. Rather than saying, "Do the vacuuming," she asks, "Can you please get the vacuuming done?" She finds that a more respectful approach works well.

Leonard is more introverted and is quieter than Barbara. He is slow to anger and thus, with Barbara being less bossy, there is little conflict in their marriage.

EDNA AND SEYMOUR

Seymour is a much more organized person than is Edna, who is more intuitive and artistic. She expresses her artistic nature in photography and ceramics. This personality difference has caused some conflict between them. Promptness is very important to Seymour. As a result, he gets angry if they are not on time, or even if they do not arrive early for an appointment. Edna believes that being on time can be rude to the host and that they should be a few minutes late. They compromise by being flexible so as to arrive close to the scheduled time.

Turning off lights is also important to Seymour. At first, Edna was somewhat casual about making sure that room lights were switched off. This behavior strikes Seymour as being wasteful. Edna believes she has overcome this habit but admits that she might slip once in a while. Seymour indicates that now if he sees an unnecessary light on, he turns it off and is silent about it. What a smart man! Some things are not worth the fuss.

Edna tends not to be as neat as Seymour. She explained, "When bringing up my children, it was more important to keep the kids happy than it was to maintain a tidy house." Seymour was used to having an uncluttered home. Now Edna tries to be neat, especially when she is working with ceramics. Seymour helps her by doing the dishes and some of the housework.

Another irritation for Seymour comes from Edna's professional training as a social worker. Seymour states, "When Edna analyzes me, it drives me nutty. She has the knack of figuring me out better than I would like, but she is usually right."

When a disagreement arises between Edna and Seymour, they sometimes become angry with each other. This can happen over "small things or little nothings that are annoying," states Edna. Seymour can become moody and introspective, signs that he wants to be left alone. The result can be a period of ignoring each other—not talking, sitting silently while watching television, or even eating meals with no discussion between them. This behavior could go on for a few days. Eventually the anger subsides and behaviors become normal again. Sometimes the silence ends with a kiss or flowers from Seymour. Often neither of them is sure why the disagreement arose in the first place. They agree that it shouldn't have been so important as to cause such dissension between them. Seymour observed, "There are things about her that irritate me and things about me that irritate her, but we work our way through them."

For me, with my need for contact, it would be almost unbearable to go several days without speaking to Jerry. But Edna is sensitive to Seymour's need to be left alone when he is upset, and this period of silence seems to work out well for them.

LAURA AND ED

Laura and Ed are somewhat similar to **Edna** and **Seymour** in their handling of conflict. Laura can blow up over something and then become completely silent for an hour or so. Ed shows anger by "clamming up" (his expression for silence) and then forgetting the issue and moving on. Like Edna and Seymour, they do not talk things out after the period of silence, but they get over their unhappiness and move on. I wonder if their ages (Laura is 80 and Ed is 90) have something to do with the lack of confrontation and no subsequent discussion. Women of Laura's generation were taught not to question their husbands; therefore "clamming up" and then dropping the matter would naturally follow.

The decision of whether to raise an issue is an individual one. If you continue to feel resentment and unhappiness, it is important to speak out when you are calm. But at times, you can decide to let the matter slide. It is good to be in touch with your own emotions and your partner's state of mind and to ask yourself, "Is this important enough for me to bring up at this time?"

KARIN AND JOHN

Karin and John have disagreements and some angry moments. Neither one displays anger openly, but each can tell when the other is displeased. This often is the case when couples are close. A tone of voice, a facial expression, or body posture can give signs to a sensitive partner that something is wrong. When Karen or John notice displeasure, one of them says, "What's troubling you?" They then talk out the disagreement, and neither holds grudges. Not holding grudges is so important. Learning to forgive and forget is a saving factor in many relationships.

CAROL AND RON

Carol and Ron have had many differences and bitter arguments during their 17 years together. They are both strong, opinionated individuals. Living together was difficult for them, and in describing their differences in how to run a home, Carol comments, "He had engineering ideas while I had aesthetic ideas." In their early days together, they would become very angry and use inappropriate words. Now that they live separately but nearby, things between them run much more smoothly. They respect each other's rules and act as a guest in the other's home.

Carol states, "It's important for me to think over a conflict situation and be cautious about how I approach the subject, depending on the outcome I want. I have learned what buttons of his to push or not to push."

Ron in turn, comments, "Sometimes she's hard on me. I know her feminist attitude. Therefore, I try to ignore small situations. Over the years, we've learned how to react to each other. We are both opinionated and independent people, but we do care for each other. In spite of differences, we help and support each other."

Indeed, over the years together, Carol and Ron have learned more positive ways of dealing with their differences, and life is much calmer and more pleasant for them now. They have grown together in their beliefs and lifestyle, learning to accept differences and to ignore less-important issues.

DOS AND DON'TS FOR HANDLING CONFLICT

These couples have many different ways of handling conflict, and each finds the way that suits them best. In this sense, there are no right or wrong ways to deal with conflict, but there are certain behaviors that are unacceptable.

First, physical violence of any kind is completely unacceptable. Women and men need to know that help is available from the police, who now receive improved training in dealing with domestic violence. Professional counseling can be beneficial. Battered women's shelters are available as a last resort. I am not aware of any shelters for battered men.

Arguments that take place under the influence of alcohol or drugs are likely to get out of hand. Control of drinking or drug use can be sought through such groups as Alcoholics Anonymous or Narcotics Anonymous.

Some simple rules for handling conflict are:

- *Do not* call each other hurtful names. Those couples interviewed who did call each other names realized they needed to stop this practice.

- *Do not* threaten to leave. This undermines the basic security of your relationship. Often when I was very angry with my late husband, I thought briefly of leaving, but I kept my mouth shut. If you are seriously thinking of ending your relationship, be sure you have a workable plan to be on your own and have first done all you can to save the partnership. Don't cry *WOLF.* Talk of leaving *only* if you really plan to do so.

- If you are very angry and the argument becomes heated, *do* take a "time out" such as leaving the room or taking a walk until you calm down. Be sure to let your partner know that you will return.

- If you are both calm and think the issue is worth talking about (you might decide some things are not important enough to discuss at all), *do* listen to your partner and really hear his or her point of view. Let him or her know that you understand, even if you do not agree. If possible, you can negotiate, each of you giving some ground. Remember, habits are hard to change, especially after having them for many years.

- *Do not* blame. Don't start a sentence with *you*, and don't use *never* or *always* such as, "You never pay attention to me." *Do* use a three-part *I* statement: (1) Name your feelings, while (2) describing in specific terms the situation that disturbs you. For example, "*I feel hurt when you look away from me as we talk.*" (3) Say concretely the change you desire. "*Please look at me when we converse, as it helps me to feel closer to you*".

- *Do not* hold grudges. *Do* forgive. Affection and humor heal many wounds.

- *Do* know that your loving relationship is more important than any small issues that bother either of you. Jerry can love me even if I leave the lights on, and I can love him even though his magazines and newspapers cover many table surfaces. He can simply turn off the lights, and I can pick up the papers and magazines. I believe that in a relationship if something small bothers you, it often is simpler and kinder to take care of it yourself rather than trying to change your partner.

IN SUMMATION

Personality differences can lead to partners complementing each other, with two different halves working together to become a harmonious whole. Some conflict is inescapable, and different styles of conflict need to be recognized and accommodated. With love, patience, humor, negotiation, and primarily, acceptance of your partner for who he or she is, an older couple can form a happy and satisfying new relationship.

Chapter 19

FRIENDSHIPS

When two young people get together, they are faced with the task of keeping old friends and developing a new friendship as a couple. Does he like her friends? Does she get along with his companions? Do they make new acquaintances together? Does either one become so involved with the new relationship that he or she neglects old friends?

These questions also apply to an older couple as they form their relationship. For older partners, friendship is often a more difficult issue. Young people make new acquaintances in both work and school environments. Parents of young children meet other parents. Retired individuals with grown children do not have the same avenues, but the need for close ties outside the primary couple's bond exists at all ages.

FRIENDS IN COMMON WHEN FIRST ACQUAINTED

Karin and **John** met while ballroom dancing. Before they became a couple, they were each in the same social circle originating from their dance club. It has been very comfortable for them to continue this association as a twosome.

Gayle and **Jim** were blessed with a lucky coincidence. The first time they met was at Gayle's art gallery. Jim went there early to meet some friends. After having an animated conversation with Gayle, his friends arrived. Surprisingly, they were also close friends of Gayle's. Jim and the friends warmly welcomed each other, to

Gayle's delight. About a month later, Gayle had a dinner party for these same friends and Jim. Their having friends in common made it so much easier for Gayle to make the first move. And so began their close relationship.

INTRODUCING FRIENDS TO YOUR NEW PARTNER

Not all couples are fortunate enough to have mutual friends before they meet. Thus, it is important to introduce your new love to your acquaintances early in your relationship. It can help reinforce your own positive assessment of your new partner and be the basis for continued association as your relationship develops.

Shortly after they met, **Ellen** took **Ralph** for a day's drive to visit close friends of hers, and he was very well accepted. This approval was important to her, as it was to me when, knowing Jerry less than a month, he joined me at a friend's home for four days, and we all got along famously. Jerry and I are still close with this couple, as are Ellen and Ralph with the friends she introduced him to.

KEEPING FRIENDS OF THE SAME SEX

It is important to maintain your closeness with friends of the same sex. This necessitates that each partner, without jealousy, allows the other separate time to maintain these ties.

Karin has a number of close women companions with whom she used to go camping. "I don't want to lose my friends," she explained, "because one danger when a woman gets involved is that she drops former associates." It is good that Karin recognizes this risk of losing old friends. She is wise to maintain her friendships.

Nancy, in her relationship with **Pat,** visits separately with intimate women friends who were part of a women's support group to which she had belonged for more than 15 years. This gives Pat, who is somewhat of a loner, his own time, and he appreciates it. Understandably, Nancy doesn't see these friends as often as before she became involved with Pat, but they are still an important part of her life.

THE CHALLENGE OF MOVING TO A NEW LOCATION

When **Mary** and **Fred** first married 20 years ago, she joined him in his home, many miles from where she had previously lived. Leaving her son and many good friends behind was a difficult adjustment. They lived in Fred's house 10 years, and it took Mary some time to feel comfortable with new acquaintances there. Then, two-and-a-half years ago, they purchased the apartment where they now live. Although this is in the same area as Mary's former home, many of her old companions had either died or moved away, so the process of making new friends was necessary.

It is interesting that Mary, not Fred, brings up their moves as adjustments. She considers herself a "people person," while Fred is more cautious in making friends. On the whole, women need more social contacts that do men, and a move can be more difficult for them. Although it took time, Mary and Fred met the challenge of finding a satisfying social life for themselves, and are now busy and happy in their present home.

THE ADVANTAGES OF RETIREMENT COMMUNITIES

The reasons for moving to retirement communities are many. Among them are wanting a warmer climate; the difficulty of keeping up the family home; escaping the crime, noise, and congestion of a city; and the inability of one or both partners to drive. For some, cooking, shopping, and house cleaning become difficult, and then moving into a community like **Mary** and **Fred's** is a godsend. It was easier for Mary and Fred to make new friends because they now live where activities are available and where all the apartments are in one building. Transportation is provided, and they take many trips to stores, restaurants, and theaters, sharing these activities with their new acquaintances. Meals are furnished, and they can chose to eat separately or with other residents. What could be more conducive to forming close relationships than dining together? **Laura** and **Ed** live in the same type of residence and also have found it relatively easy to make new friends.

Edna and **Seymour** reside in a large retirement community where many homes are spread over much acreage. Many activities are offered, but they cook their own meals and provide their own transportation for trips outside the community. They play bridge with other couples and invite each other for dinners. They have acquaintances with whom they garden, make ceramics, and play golf. They have lived in the community four years and gradually, from these shared activities, have made many good friends.

It is not merely the shared activities that create close friendships. Jerry and I are both active in our rural community, but we have made more casual acquaintances than true friends. Most of the people we meet have lived in our area for many years and have their own well-developed social circles. Although they are very friendly, they do not reach out for new, close ties. In a retirement community, many of the residents are initially in the same boat; fairly newly arrived and searching for friendship. Thus, though a move to a retirement community has the disadvantage of extending distance from old friends, it has the advantage of making it much easier to form new, close associations.

THE BENEFITS OF STAYING PUT

Mary Pipher, in her interesting book, *Another Country* (Riverhead Books, 1999), is a passionate advocate of the older adult remaining in his or her own community, near family and old friends, and with an opportunity to know individuals of all generations. She particularly stresses how, in moving away, many older adults lose frequent contact with their children and grandchildren. She writes, "We want the generations to mix together so that the young can give the old joy and the old can give the young wisdom" (page 322). I heed Pipher's admonition. I have a three-hour drive to my daughter's home and hope not to move farther from her at any future time.

Karin and **John,** and **Joanne** and **Andy** have remained in their earlier locations. John's cousin lives nearby. He and John run together regularly, and John and Karin socialize with John's cousin and his wife. They also have other old friends in the same community with whom they spend time as couples. They are both particularly close to Karin's best friend and her partner.

Joanne, dwelling in the same area since childhood, has many friends and still spends time with them. Andy is near his daughter, who visits their home often. She and Joanne have become close.

Although a move to a retirement community may bring many built-in activities, living in a city or a small town offers many diversions as long as one can walk, bike, or drive to them. My previous community, near my daughter, offered many theater and restaurant options, a senior exercise class, and an Olympic-size swimming pool, all only a five-minute drive or a short walk from my home.

A move may become necessary when, among other reasons, one or both partners become unable to drive. In this case however, children, grandchildren, or friends often are able to visit frequently and to help with transportation.

Though it is certainly possible to make friends in a new location, remaining near old friends may be more advantageous. A recent study emphasizes how lengthy friendships contribute to the positive self-image of older adults.

"Aging adults seek friends who can reduce the discrepancy between their perception of who they are and the negative identity meanings they might receive from family and others" ("Friendship and Social Support: The Importance of Role Identity to Aging Adults," *Social Work*, November 1999, page 529).

As the older adult becomes more dependent, he or she might be treated with less regard by family or recent acquaintances. The old friend who knew him or her during more productive years is more likely to relate in a manner that reinforces the earlier, more positive self-image.

My dearest friend visited me recently. We are both psychotherapists and still have much respect for each other professionally, often consulting on difficult cases. We had much fun reminiscing about backpacking and river-rafting adventures that we enjoyed together in the past, and which neither of us is physically able to do now. Thus, we reinforced each other's present-day positive self-identity.

RELIGIOUS INSTITUTIONS AS FRIENDSHIP SOURCES

Donna and **Stuart**, living in their own home in a rural community, are very active in their church. They enjoy many potlucks with friends there, and their church is their primary social group. Donna smiles when saying, "I've been accepted so well in Stuart's church. We've made many good friends since I've joined. They are a great support for Stuart and me."

Edna and **Seymour,** and **Naomi** and **David**, reside in retirement communities and are active in their synagogues where they have made many good friends. A religious congregation welcomes newcomers and in addition to services, offers many congenial activities. This subject is covered in more detail in Chapter 20, *Religious Beliefs and Practices.*

WHEN OLD FRIENDS DIE

One problem with living to a ripe old age is that many good friends die first. Such losses can lead to isolation and depression. Being with a loving partner can help greatly. In our study, three of the men, **Fred**, **Cliff**, and **David** have lost close friends. None of the three has replaced these companions with others as intimate. Fred's friends had been part of his working life, and he grew apart from them after retirement. David was used to doing things with other men, and now that he is unable to fish or play golf, he is no longer in contact with them. He still has one good friend who is living, but neither of them is well enough to visit the other. Instead, they talk on the phone frequently. Although friends have died, Cliff still has close ties with his 10 brothers. He is lucky to have 10 built-in male companions.

Losing close friends through death seems to happen more frequently to men, because men generally die younger than do women. And as men tend to have fewer close ties, the loss can be more severe. I remember when, several years ago, a man I was close to died suddenly of a heart attack. His best friend, who lived 3,000 miles away, was grief stricken. They had seen action together during World War II, and their strong emotional bond had lasted all these years. He believed he would never again have such a close relationship; certainly the ties men form during wartime are almost irreplaceable.

I lost one of my dearest friends several years ago. We had been very close in New York City when we were both in our twenties. After I moved to California, I saw her only on the rare occasions when I traveled East. During the last few years of her life, I knew she had cancer, and we had infrequent phone contacts. The cancer kept reappearing, but she always sounded upbeat and hopeful. I was in denial. I never fully realized she was going to die. Then one day I received a letter from her sister informing me that she had died after several months in a nursing home. I was distraught. Mostly, I regretted that I had not kept in better touch and had not gone to see her when she was ill.

I learned from this experience. This past year another friend, in the Netherlands, was in a hospital, soon to die of cancer. I flew to Holland and had a brief emotional visit with her. The next day she died. I am so glad we had a chance to say goodbye. It was much more important for me to visit while she was still alive than to attend her funeral.

It is vital to keep in touch with close friends from many years past—more than the yearly Christmas letter. That way you can more accurately ascertain the state of your friend's health and be there when needed. Jerry has a good friend who is gradually going downhill with prostate cancer. He visits and phones him frequently. Jerry hopes he will have the opportunity to say goodbye when the time comes.

With cancer there is a chance to bid farewell. This is not so with a sudden heart attack. Still, if you have been in fairly close contact, you should be less regretful about opportunities lost. Grieving is less painful if it is without guilt or remorse. When a good friend dies, take comfort in memories of your times together and in the joys of your present life.

MEN AND FRIENDSHIPS

Most of the men I interviewed had far fewer intimate friends that did their mates. All however, appreciated joining their partners' social circle.

Joanne has many friends with whom she spends time. During the nine years that **Andy** was unattached, he joined singles clubs, and his only friends were women. He no longer feels comfortable associating with them now that he is in a relationship with Joanne. "I guess I didn't bother much with men friends those days after my divorce. Now I wish I had," says Andy. At present, Andy enjoys Joanne's acquaintances, and recently he had asked her to invite mutual friends to a dinner party to celebrate his birthday.

Nancy has more intimate friends than does **Pat.** He told me he has just his large family and Nancy. "Nancy's the only friend I need," he explained. They are close with a few couples who were originally Nancy's friends.

Carol has many friends from where she previously lived, and they visit each other for as much as a week at a time. **Ron** has few friends but enjoys getting together with Carol's acquaintances. He prefers working around the house and in the garden during the day and then reading and watching television in the evening.

Like Ron, Jerry is content to work in our orchard during the day and then to spend quiet evenings at home. In many ways, this is an advantage and I marvel at how self-sufficient he is. Many of the men I interviewed are equally content to be at home, either alone or with their partners.

My late husband had only one close man friend, a sailing companion. Early in our marriage, he often spoke to me of missing the friendship of men. Eventually, he joined a small weekly men's group. When he first heard of such a gathering, he wondered what activities they participated in. Did they bowl or go fishing? He couldn't imagine that men could just sit around and talk, sharing experiences, problems, and accomplishments. For many years however, until his death, this small group of men was a central part of his life. Such a group is leaderless and not difficult to form. I strongly recommend to men readers that if they miss the close friendship of other men, they consider forming such a group. With my first husband, the friendship of these men greatly enriched his life, thereby benefiting our relationship.

IN SUMMATION

Each person has a different need for close companionship. As we grow older, we lose friends through illness and death. Moving to a new community can mean the loss of old friends and gradually the acquisition of new acquaintances. Retirement communities bring together many older people who may be eager to form new ties. For some, staying in the area where they have lived for many years means keeping active the connections with family and friends. When one member of a couple is well established, the new partner often moves into a ready-made social circle.

For both partners, when the union is a good one, the joy of being with each other can outweigh any difficulties incurred in forming new friendships. But no two people, no matter how much they are in love, are an island unto themselves. Pleasure can be found by spending time with other couples. Individual friendships help to keep the necessary balance of separateness and togetherness in a relationship. Without doubt, establishing and maintaining genuine friendships remain vital to the older couple, newly coupled.

Chapter 20

RELIGIOUS BELIEFS AND PRACTICES

Religion offers many benefits to the faithful. Membership in a religious congregation provides a sense of community and a social life, while members support each other through difficult times. Belief in God and an afterlife greatly helps when facing hardship and death. Research shows that religion assists individuals to live longer. One large study followed more than 5,000 Californians for 28 years. Those who attended religious services at least once a week had a 23 percent lower risk of dying during the study period than those who attended less frequently, even after the researchers controlled for lifestyle factors and social support (*Journal of Public Health,* June 1997, page 48).

Many of those interviewed for this book belong to a church or a temple, and for some, religion is a central aspect of their lives. On the other hand, those who have no religious associations seem to do well in their lives, with other ethical convictions and activities sustaining them. Among our couples, affiliations include fundamentalist Christian, mainstream Protestant, Catholic, and Jewish faiths. While most believe in God and an afterlife, some are agnostic. Beliefs also include reincarnation, the Goddess religion, and the importance of humanitarian values. While many of the individuals interviewed came from the same or similar denominations as their partner, others held different belief systems but were respectful of each other's religious views. Let us examine this very important aspect of newly coupled, older couples' lives.

STUART AND DONNA

Before their marriage, Stuart and Donna were members of different conservative Christian congregations. In the beginning stages of their relationship, Stuart expressed concern that Donna was of a different denomination, but their religious beliefs were not that far apart. Stuart's Christian and moral convictions made him acceptable to Donna. Then during their courtship together, they attended services at each other's churches.

Their religious beliefs caused them to refrain from sexual intercourse until after marriage. Once married, Donna converted to Stuart's church. They are both very active in this congregation, which shapes the major activity of their social life. Their church is active worldwide and takes care of its members in many ways. In his will, Stuart is leaving his house, not to Donna or to his children, but to his church. In return, he sees no need for long-term-care insurance as he knows his church will take care of him and Donna, should it be needed.

RUTH AND PAUL

All members of Paul's family were faithful participants in a minority Christian group. As a child, he was teased because of his religion, but it remained important to him, and he continues to worship in a local church of that same denomination. He is active in its congregation, and it is an important part of his life.

Ruth had shifted from one Christian belief to another during her youth and through her first marriage. Now she attends services at her husband's church but has not joined the congregation because she believes she has her own religion. She believes in the Golden Rule and in the teachings of Jesus Christ, recognizing "the wonders of this wonderful world that God has given us."

EDNA AND SEYMOUR

Seymour is Jewish and feels strongly about practicing his faith. He has a firm allegiance to Israel, where a sister lives and where his parents are buried. For years he was active in a Conservative congregation, but the temple he and Edna attend in their retirement community is Reform and has no permanent rabbi.

Edna describes herself as an agnostic. She believes in living by the Golden Rule: "Do unto others as you would have them do unto you." Edna also believes in past lives and what can be learned about people from studying their astrological signs. She seldom discusses these beliefs with Seymour. Although he doesn't share her beliefs, he respects her right to hold them.

Seymour had a brief, unsuccessful marriage after he had already become involved with Edna. It was based on the fact that the woman he so hastily married was Jewish. In returning to Edna, he accepted the differences in their belief systems, and by mutual respect, they made a smooth adjustment to these differences.

Seymour is active with Jewish groups in the community. Edna would convert, but Seymour doesn't believe it is important for her to do so. She participates in religious services and finds the moral, caring beliefs of Judaism readily acceptable to her. In accordance with these convictions, they both work in a shelter for the homeless that is under the auspices of a Jewish organization.

Edna and Seymour's recognition of each other's traditions is exemplified by their celebration of Christmas, Hanukkah, Passover, and Easter. All generations gather to celebrate these holidays, showing a wholesome acceptance of each other's heritages. At Hanukkah and Christmas time, gifts are exchanged, but no Christmas tree is on exhibit. The tree was important in Edna's childhood, but it is unacceptable to Seymour. Instead, Hanukkah candles in a menorah (an eight-branched candelabrum) are displayed to symbolize the eight days of the festival of Hanukkah.

Edna and Seymour's situation brings to mind that of good friends of ours. The husband, like Seymour, is Jewish and strong in his faith. His wife comes from a Scandinavian Christian background. She participates with her husband in temple activities and religious celebrations, but like Edna, has not converted to her husband's religion. I have attended many wonderful seders (the feast of Passover) in their home. Their main conflict revolves around the Christmas tree, which holds important memories for the wife from her childhood. The tree is unacceptable to her husband, and recently they have resolved this problem by traveling during the holidays. My friends, along with Edna and Seymour, are inspiring examples of how mutual respect for each other's beliefs can enhance a relationship.

MARY AND FRED

Mary and Fred, like Edna and Seymour, are another couple from different denominational backgrounds but who respect each other's beliefs. Fred was raised Catholic and Mary Protestant. They each attend their own church and sometimes go to each other's services. Both believe that religion is essential "to keep people fair and honest."

NANCY AND PAT

Both Pat and Nancy are Catholic and became acquainted through their church. Pat doesn't consider himself as strong a Catholic as Nancy is, but he goes to church every Sunday to be with her. His late wife was also a devout Catholic and he went to church with her. He jocularly states, "Nancy's going to get me into Heaven one way or the other. She prays for me. I can't miss. All I have to do is be nice to Nancy from now on and not kick the dog." (Neither one has a dog!)

Nancy and Pat are not married. I asked Nancy how her relationship with Pat has been accepted by their congregation and how it fits with her religious convictions. Nancy tells me that they walk into church every Sunday holding hands. No one has ever said anything, and she hasn't offered any explanation. She told me, "Our partnership is so right. The whole purpose of love is the ultimate sharing. We haven't hurt anyone. We don't have to worry about birth control. I have not talked with anyone about our relationship from a spiritual point of view, because I know it's right for me. It's our conscience that is the ultimate guide. We take care of each other, and we make each other so happy. We're committed."

NAOMI AND DAVID

Naomi and David are another example of a couple for whom religion is central to their lives—in this instance, Judaism. They are both active in their Reform temple and in the past, David had been a cantor, singing during services.

David and Naomi met at a temple service. Naomi's paintings of the Torah and of a rabbi adorn their walls, while a mezuzah hangs on their entrance door. (The mezuzah is a small piece of parchment inscribed with a quote from the Old Testament, enclosed in metal, and attached to the doorpost of a home, as commanded in the Biblical passages).

David was raised in an orthodox Jewish orphanage where he learned Hebrew. Naomi's parents belonged to the Workmen's Circle, a Jewish Socialist group. Through involvement with this group, she learned to read and write Hebrew fluently. While she read stories and histories of the Jewish people, she wasn't taught to believe in God. Today she believes that there might be a God.

CAROL AND RON

Carol had few religious experiences as a youth or during her marriages. Ron was brought up as an Episcopalian, but he did not continue to observe his faith in later life.

Now they both have a strong interest in a nondenominational religious philosophy and together attend a church espousing this philosophy while honoring all deities. As Ron explained, "What we have now follows beliefs I have held most of my life. Each person is in control of what happens to him or her. If the person thinks positively about something, it will happen. You are what you believe, and you can be able to do whatever you want. The responsibility for beliefs and actions rests with each individual."

Carol also has become very involved with these concepts. She attends a *Positive Living Center* with Ron. Previously, she considered herself an atheist. Now she reads about religions extensively and strongly believes in self-healing and psychic phenomena.

GAYLE AND JIM

Gayle, as a child, was baptized Episcopalian, while Jim considers himself a "recovering Catholic." Now they both attend, as do **Carol** and **Ron**, a *Positive Living Center* that portends, "If you relate to the world with a positive attitude, it affects how you function and what life means to you."

Gayle, a feminist, also is a devotee of the Goddess religion. When she was hoping to find the right man, she prayed under a full moon to her Goddess for help. (Goddess-worshipping religions flourished in Europe between 6500 and 3500 BC. At that time it is believed that there was no warfare and that peaceful societies were guided by a priestess-queen.)

JOANNE AND ANDY

Like Nancy and Pat, Joanne and Andy were raised Catholic. The difference is that they do not practice this religion. It was their being "strayed Catholics" that attracted them to each other. Their similar religious upbringings and their falling away from the church was part of what bonded them. Both are still influenced by their upbringing, keeping much of their faith and belief in a Divine Being and an afterlife.

JANICE AND CLIFF

Janice was raised Catholic, while Cliff's family attended the Lutheran church. At present, neither one is involved with any particular religion, but they are searching. Janice wants a spiritual connection because both she and Cliff are "fairly spiritual, believing in God." She also believes in reincarnation and karma ("If you do good in the world, what goes around, comes around"). In her own words, "We all have responsibilities to the planet and to other people living here." Janice believes strongly that she and Cliff had "been together in a previous life." They both believe in having lives previous to the present ones.

Cliff shares Janice's views by being open about religions, believing in forgiveness, tolerance, and accepting alternative lifestyles. He prefers hearing church sermons having intellectual substance, and has attended various churches during holiday periods to learn about their message and what needs they serve in the community.

OTHER NON-ATTENDING COUPLES

Like **Joanne** and **Andy,** and **Janice** and **Cliff,** other couples interviewed do not attend any church or temple. **Barbara** and **Leonard** describe themselves as agnostic, although Barbara strongly believes that her friends' prayers helped her recover from cancer.

Laura and **Ed**, while not attending church, do watch services on television. Ed has had many severe medical problems, so this procedure for recognizing religion is understandable.

Other non-attending couples include those who are not sure there is a God, but all are caring individuals, and lead good lives.

IN SUMMATION

All the individuals interviewed have found their own unique paths to the kinds of worship, or non-worship, that suit them. Some couples are solidly together in their beliefs, attending the same church. Others have different religious affiliations but respect this dissimilarity in the same way that they recognize and honor other differences between themselves. This togetherness in faith, or a tolerance of dissimilar beliefs, contributes to a successful partnership when older couples are newly coupled.

Chapter 21

MONETARY AND LEGAL ARRANGEMENTS, Including Thoughts about the End of Life

This chapter treats financial and legal arrangements made by the couples interviewed. The financial decisions are divided into two parts. One is how to share ongoing expenses, including house payments, utilities, food, entertainment, and travel. The other part deals with specifying how and to whom assets are left after death. Here, legal instruments such as wills, trusts, and premarital agreements come into play. (See Chapter 26 for descriptions of these instruments.)

As I discussed legal matters with our couples, we also considered whether the woman had changed her name and whether the couple may have made decisions about purchasing long-term-care insurance. Finally, attitudes toward the end of life were explored, including whether to extend life in the event of a terminal illness. All these concerns are examined in this chapter.

ONGOING EXPENSES

The decision about how to share expenses often is made early in the courtship, especially when it comes to entertainment. This agreement then extends to all living expenses as the couple becomes more deeply involved. For couples who live separately, this matter is less complicated, as household expenses are not involved.

Nancy and **Pat,** who are unmarried but very much committed to each other, are an example of such a couple. They live separately in two identical small apartments in a retirement community. Each pays his or her own home expenses, and the host or hostess provides the meals when they visit each other's apartments. When they go out, they take turns treating each other, and when traveling, they split all expenses.

Karin and **John** also are not married and live separately. Karin is better off financially than is John, and she is perfectly content with this difference. John takes some food when he stays at her home, although she provides most of it. John thinks it would be easier if they were living together and he could pay something toward her townhouse expenses. He wants to live with Karin, but she is hesitant.

Karin must battle with John in order to pay her share of dinners, movies, and other entertainment, because he wants to pay it all. This must be a matter of masculine pride. It has long been the custom for the man to treat when a couple goes out, and being the partner with less money might be difficult for John. The circumstances in which the difference in their financial status could be a problem is with vacations, as Karin can afford more expensive trips than can John. As a solution, they plan to travel as reasonably as possible, and Karin accepts it that way.

Joanne and **Andy** are unmarried, living together, and Joanne is still actively consulting in her field, while Andy is retired. Despite Joanne's income being greater than Andy's, they share equally. With Andy, Joanne enjoys the sharing of all expenses. While they have separate checking accounts, they split the rent and utilities equally and put money in a basket to use for food and household expenses. Like **Karin** and **John**, the only time they anticipate difficulties with this difference in income is when they travel.

David and **Naomi, Laura** and **Ed,** and **Ellen** and **Ralph** are three married couples who share their living expenses equally.

Because Naomi has considerably more financial resources than does David, she bought their present home in a retirement community, and she pays the maintenance expenses for this home. To equalize matters, David pays for food and utilities, and they split travel and entertainment expenses.

Ellen and **Ralph** use the same method. When they lived in Ralph's apartment, he paid the home expenses, and Ellen took care of all groceries, the phone, and other living expenses. They now live and travel in a recreational vehicle that they bought together with their accumulated savings and the proceeds from the sale of Ralph's home.

Laura and **Ed** have a slight variation in handling expenses. They put the same amount monthly into a joint checking account for all their expenses, but Laura reimburses this account for personal expenses such as clothing.

Mary and **Fred**, a married couple, are an example of the man having the major income to handle expenses. Mary has a small income from her Social Security benefits that is kept in a separate bank account and which she uses for her personal needs. Mary, at 85 years of age, spent most of her adult life as a housewife, raising her son. It is fortunate that now she has some funds of her own to give her a degree of independence. When the man holds the purse strings, it is sometimes he who has more power in the relationship. This appears to be the case with Mary and Fred and also with **Donna** and **Stuart**.

Mary and **Fred**, and **Donna** and **Stuart** might have more traditional values than do the other couples interviewed, for not all of the individuals who are financially better off hold more power in their relationship. An example is **Ruth** and **Paul**, as Paul is wealthier than Ruth, yet they equally divide expenses and decision-making. Ruth owns the home in which they live, and they split their utility and home-maintenance charges. Paul pays the larger bills for purchases, travel, and dining out, while Ruth handles the costs for groceries.

Gayle and **Jim** are a younger couple, who are living together, though not married. Gayle is better off financially than is Jim. Gayle owns the house and the property where they live. Jim, because of previous debts, handles only the utilities and the telephone bills, while Gayle pays for food and travel expenses. As long as Jim works freelance, Gayle encourages him to put any excess income he has into investments to benefit himself. Gayle manages their financial accounts. This is an artistic couple with new-age beliefs, and they are both comfortable with the woman being the older and wealthier partner.

CONFLICTS OVER SPENDING

It is important to look at different attitudes about spending. With **Laura** and **Ed**, a major issue, according to Laura, relates to Ed's perceived frugality in spending money. Laura likes to buy some things on the spur of the moment, and Ed often thinks this is frivolous. His attitude might be due to his upbringing during the Depression of the 1930s. While Laura has money of her own, and their sharing of expenses is equal, there is still some conflict between them when she buys something expensive with her own money.

Since differences in spending money within any relationship may lead to arguments, I analyzed this matter further with Laura and Ed. With her first husband, Laura made many decisions on her own about purchasing things for the house. This was okay with her husband. On the other hand, Ed and his first wife planned their purchases together. Thus, this aspect of Laura and Ed's previous spending patterns differ, and the behaviors are carried over into their present relationship, resulting in some disagreements.

Couples need to look at previous patterns to better understand and accept present differences. After their talk with me about their previous spending patterns, this understanding helped Laura and Ed. Laura buys what she wants, and with their mutual acceptance of dissimilar views, any disagreement is short-lived.

Ruth and **Paul** are another example of different attitudes about money. In this case, the wife is more frugal than her husband. Paul is more affluent than Ruth; thus he is accustomed to spending money more freely. Here are two examples of their different attitudes. As a result of Paul's past business experience, he uses the telephone a great deal and makes lengthy calls. This bothers Ruth. At first they took turns paying the telephone bill, but now if a bill is excessive, Paul pays the extra amount. Paul often allows lights to continue burning after he leaves a room. Ruth reminds him of this, but he often forgets. She now turns the lights off without comment, and he pays excessively high utility charges. By taking responsibility for added telephone and light costs, Paul has diffused conflict with Ruth. She is still free to hold her belief regarding the spending of money. She says, "By living through the Depression years of the 1930s, my generation learned the value of a dollar, and we are still careful with our purchases."

INHERITANCE

Our couples vary as to whom they leave their assets. Some will money and property to each other. Others, knowing their partners are financially self-sufficient, provide inheritances for their children and grandchildren.

Assets Left to Children

Nancy and **Pat** each has a living trust that leaves assets to their children. **Karin** and **John** also have arranged inheritances for their children. Karin has a will, leaving all of her assets to her children and grandchildren. John has no trust or will, as there would be little to divide among his children. He believes that they will manage matters involving the sharing of his limited estate without conflict.

Laura and **Ed** have a premarital agreement and separate trusts, providing that assets acquired before their marriage stay with each individual and are inherited by each one's daughter and grandchildren.

Though **Bill** has established a living trust, leaving his assets to his children, he is putting aside a percentage of his investments for **Joyce** in case he dies first. It is encouraging that despite their difficult relationship, Bill wants to help Joyce with her future financial security.

Assets Left to Each Other

Some couples leave their assets primarily to each other rather than to their children. **Mary** and **Fred** name each other as primary inheritors, using a prenuptial agreement, separate wills, and living trusts. After both of their deaths, their assets will pass proportionately to each one's daughter and on to their grandchildren.

Carol and **Ron** also have established living trusts, leaving their assets to each other. Carol has no children, and Ron has one daughter. Ron feels certain that his greater income would comfortably take care of Carol, should he die first because her own funds are decreasing. Ron's daughter would be the heir in his will after Carol, and he has left her a small proportion of his estate upon his death.

Ellen and **Ralph** also name each other as beneficiaries. Each one has established a living trust and a will for this purpose. Ellen does not think that her children will need her money, while Ralph believes it is more important to leave assets to Ellen than to his children. This is an example of how each considers their own relationship primary and that with their children secondary. It fits with the lack of acceptance of the marriage by Ralph's children and Ellen's limited contact with her three children.

Three of the women have given their partners the right to remain in their homes even though the properties eventually will pass to their children. Each has arranged this differently.

Naomi, through her living trust, allows **David** to remain in the house and provides that the first $600,000 will be divided among her children and grandchildren; the rest will be left to **David** until he dies.

Janice and **Cliff** have established a postnuptial agreement that passes on their assets as stated in each of their wills. Janice has an interesting way of dividing her funds after her death. Her brother, as trustee, will distribute her estate according to the needs of the inheritors, but her will allows Cliff to remain in the house until his death.

Barbara has used a prenuptial agreement to ensure that upon her death, **Leonard** may continue to live in the house as long as he wishes before her daughter acquires it.

THE WOMAN'S NAME CHANGE

This matter can be a part of legal arrangements after marriage. Whether a woman changes her name to her husband's depends greatly upon the woman's outlook on life and her sense of identity.

Donna, a very traditional Christian lady, not only changed her name without question, but very much resents being addressed by mail as *Ms* rather than *Mrs.*

Laura, Mary, Ruth, and **Naomi** all have taken their husband's names. **Barbara** has kept all of her property in her former name, but has changed the surname on her driver's license and Social Security account. **Ellen** has been phasing out her previous surname for personal use, business matters, and on legal documents, replacing it with her new, married name. Ellen's extra effort in changing her name shows her basic traditional outlook despite the fact that she is very independent as a businesswoman

Two of the women decided not to change their names. **Carol** has kept her maiden name and does not use **Ron's** surname in any way. This is acceptable to Ron. **Janice** has kept her maiden surname, which she re-established after her divorce. It is the name she has used in her professional life and she still uses it for identifications on her driver's license, bank account, and Social Security account. For some purposes, she uses this name hyphenated with **Cliff's** surname, but mostly it is important to her sense of identity to keep her maiden name. Cliff accepts all of her decisions about name use.

Like Janice, my own name use is a compromise. I have kept my previous married name, *Ankersmit,* on all identifying documents and investments. Keeping this name is particularly important to me professionally. I often use *Ankersmit Kemp,* as shown on the title page of this book. Socially I respond to *Edith Kemp.*

POWER OF ATTORNEY FOR HEALTH CARE

This is an important document that each individual should complete. It specifies your wishes regarding being kept alive in the event of a terminal illness and who has the right to make this decision. For unmarried couples, this form is essential, as without this document, neither individual would have any say regarding his or her partner's medical treatment. See page 325 for additional information.

Nancy does not want to be kept alive unnaturally and has completed this form, although her partner, **Pat** has not done so. **Barbara** and **Leonard** have signed Power of Attorney for Healthcare forms so that each can make life-support decisions for the other. In the document, Barbara's daughter and Leonard's son follow each of them with the decision-making power.

Janice and **Cliff** also have completed this form. Janice is the executor for Cliff, and her brother is her executor. Neither wants "any medical heroics" in the event one or the other becomes terminally ill. They will donate any usable organs to an appropriate organization.

While **Laura** and **Ed** have not prepared the Power of Attorney for Health Care forms, they both have understandings with their children about limiting their terminal care. After our discussion, they agreed to consider completing such a document, as it would ensure better legal compliance with their wishes.

LONG-TERM-CARE INSURANCE

The pros and cons of acquiring long-term-care insurance are discussed in Chapter 26. Our couples vary in assessing the need for this insurance. Age, health, and financial circumstances have contributed to their decisions.

Pat has long-term-care insurance, while his partner, **Nancy**, does not. Pat does not want to burden his children with his care. He is aware that, with his failing eyesight, if Nancy dies first, he may need assistance. Nancy is in good health and believes that it is unlikely that she will require extended nursing-home care.

Naomi has provided this insurance for **David,** who already is suffering serious health problems and memory loss. But he says, "I'm not going to need it." He does not want to think of this eventuality. How few of us do. Naomi does not believe that she needs such insurance, as she has sufficient assets to cover her care.

Both **Barbara and Leonard** have long-term-care insurance, having purchased it separately at a younger age when it was less expensive for them. They do not want their children to be forced to care for them.

Both **Gayle** and **Jim** have long-term-care insurance. A financial planner recommended it to Gayle. She acquired it through her deceased husband's company plan. Jim also has this insurance because at his younger age, it seemed inexpensive.

Laura and **Ed,** ages 80 and 90, believe this insurance is too expensive for consideration at their advanced ages. The reader needs to determine his or her own perceived need for this insurance against whatever the cost might be.

ATTITUDES TOWARD THE END OF LIFE

All of our couples know that their time together is limited and precious. The title of **Joanne** and **Andy's** interview chapter, "*Life is Short, Eat Dessert First,*" exemplifies this belief. Attitudes of our couples toward eventual death differ.

Nancy and **Pat** are very aware of their increasing ages and have discussed both illness and death. Nancy, who did volunteer hospice work in the past, has been trained to accept death. She and Pat wonder who will go first. Pat laughed and said, "I hope it will be in the middle of sex," and then he continued seriously, "One of us is going to be alone. Living in this retirement community will be helpful at that time." He thinks Nancy will be the better survivor, as she is more practical and better organized.

Carol and **Ron** have discussed this topic together. In Ron's words, "I'm ready. I will not be in control when that time comes, and whatever is, will be. But I believe I'll come back at a later time." (This is a belief in reincarnation, part of Hindu and Buddhist belief systems.) Carol thinks she will die before Ron. Why? "Because Ron is a long-termer."

Carol believes in near-death experiences that indicate that there is an afterlife. She is not fearful of death. She states, "The soul leaves the body and is transported to another world." This gives her a strong desire to make sure that Ron's body is handled properly when he dies; in her words, "so he is not mistreated when he passes on to another world."

When asked about whether she thinks at all about death, **Laura** says, "It does enter my mind," while **Ed** says, "It doesn't frighten me." They agree that "time is running out, and we never know who will go first."

When the subject of death was raised, **Gayle** indicated that she thinks of it frequently. This is because of the sudden death of her husband and the injuries **Jim** received in a car accident while she was driving. Gayle expects to live to age 100 because many of her relatives lived into their late 90s. Gayle and Jim each express concern about the other one dying first and the sorrow this would create. Gayle, with her spiritual beliefs, states humorously, knowing she is a bit bossy, "When I die, I will return as an angel, sit on people's shoulders, and tell them what to do."

When asked about facing the end of life, **Mary** prays that she will go first, while **Fred** said, "If life becomes more pain than pleasure, I want to go and have no one stop me. I'll probably request sleeping tablets from my doctor." This brings up the controversy of assisted suicide, at present illegal in all states but Oregon. Unless laws change, Fred would not be able to get a large quantity of sleeping pills from his doctor.

Paul and **Ruth** have a somewhat different attitude toward death. Paul, smiling, said, "Maybe we'll both live to 100. It would be a shame to quit sooner when we are so close." Ruth, smiling, nodded her head in agreement.

Cliff has an outlook similar to Paul's. He does not think much about death. In his words, "Life is too full to really be concerned with death. But when it does come, I'll not be fearful of it." **Janice** indicated that she thinks about the end of life because her parents are aging, and close friends have recently died. This discussion caused her to again express her regrets about not having had children. Janice and Cliff both would like to die together. Cliff expresses the concern, "What would happen to me if Janice goes first?" Janice, like Ron, believes in reincarnation. When Janice hears certain music, she thinks about how nice it would be to use it at her funeral.

Barbara and **Leonard** said that they talk about death and an afterlife at times, but Barbara stated, "I don't want to even think about death. We're not concerned with who goes first, and we'll face things as they come. I don't want to cross this bridge until necessary."

Leonard agreed, "Me too ... that's the best way."

Paul, Ruth, Cliff, Leonard, and Barbara exemplify the attitude that life in the present is too full and happy to spend much time thinking about death. Despite their older age and the knowledge that life ends sooner or later, they feel young, and death seems far away. Since I've been with Jerry, despite my years, I feel inside like a young girl in love. I know someday we each will die, but I hope it will be many years from now.

Our couples, by their preparation of wills and trusts, have acknowledged in a practical way the inevitability of death. For some, thoughts of life ending are very much in mind. Others do not wish to contemplate death, focusing, rather on present joys. For most, beliefs and attitudes about eventual death are an essential part of their perspectives on life.

IN SUMMATION

Money management is a crucial ingredient in any union, and partners work out what suits them best. A City Bank survey finds that "57% of all divorces stem from arguments over money" (*Time* magazine, June 25, 1999, page 80). This statistic emphasizes how important it is to be clear with your partner about how expenses are shared and to whom resources are willed.

Each of our couples has their own unique way of sharing expenses and providing inheritances. They also vary in their thoughts about the end of life and in making decisions concerning name change, Power of Attorney for Health Care, and long-term-care insurance.

We recommend that you consider our couples' experiences and discuss alternatives with your partner so that by sharing these important and personal matters, your relationship will become closer and stronger.

Section Three

HOW DO YOU FIND A PARTNER?

This Section is designed for older, single individuals who are seeking a companion. Unless you are fortunate enough to meet someone you like by chance, it is necessary to make a concerted effort to find a person who interests you. Here you will find answers to these questions:

Many of the suggestions in these chapters are illustrated by the experiences of our couples, with their names appearing in **boldface**. When appropriate, Edith adds comments from both her professional and personal knowledge.

Chapter 22

ARE YOU READY?

Being ready is as much within your heart as it is within your head. Real readiness is something you gradually come to recognize. The ultimate question, on both a head and heart level, is, *"How ready are you for commitment and intimacy?"* Reading this book may be your first step toward an answer.

Many persons talk about wanting to meet someone of the opposite sex, and some may be emotionally prepared to start the search process. For others, their actions do not go beyond words because, on an unconscious level, something is holding them back. Others may rush too quickly into their search for a partner, and this could lead to forming an unsatisfactory relationship.

HASTY ACTION

Hasty action could take place shortly after a divorce or after the death of a spouse. In one's anxiety to find someone to fill the gap in his or her life, clues often can be overlooked that ordinarily would be noticed. For example, **Seymour** married quite soon after his wife's death. He saw only the externals. The woman was of his religion and was wealthy. He failed to recognize that she had a drinking problem and that there was no comfortable camaraderie between them. Ordinarily, it is possible to notice the signs of excessive drinking, and if we listen to our feelings, we know if we are comfortable and happy with a companion. But in his urgency,

Seymour ignored these clues, and the marriage lasted only a few months.

In another situation, **Ralph** lost his first wife to breast cancer after six years of marriage. Within six months he married a woman 16 years younger than himself. In Ralph's words, "This was a big mistake. She married me for my money. She disliked my kids and they hated her. It was stupid on my part." Ralph divorced her after only four months.

Bob, a good friend of my husband, Jerry, had an experience similar to those of Seymour and Ralph. After 36 years of marriage and many years of a sex life that was infrequent and with limited pleasure, his wife died. He was longing for love, companionship, and sexual fulfillment. About six months after his wife's death, he contacted a dating service of his religion. Through it he met a woman who was extremely attractive and lived an impressive lifestyle (in a big city no less, while Bob is a country boy). He was completely blinded, swept off his feet, and they were married at her insistence, within a few months. They had completely different lifestyles. Bob was not happy living in her city apartment and she despised his country home and way of life there. Her extravagant lifestyle and insistence that he pay all her expenses cost him a great deal financially. They had frequent, bitter arguments and marriage counseling was of no help. Bob left her and initiated a divorce three months after the marriage. He has since learned that friends and family who met her wondered how he could have picked someone with whom he was so poorly matched. Some had hinted their concern to him, but most were reluctant to say anything.

Bob, like Seymour and Ralph, reacted very quickly after his wife's death by remarrying and never asked the question posed in this chapter: *Are you ready*? He just jumped into deep water, came to the surface before drowning, and revived to an eventual good life with another wife. He painfully learned an important lesson!

ONCE THE GRIEVING IS OVER

Ralph, **Seymour**, and Bob were, in a way, fortunate. They were able to end their hasty marriages quickly. Others, both men and women, may still be living unhappily in marriages they made too soon after a painful loss. You need to be sure you are not merely running from grief, or from a fear of being alone, in seeking a new love after losing your mate. On the other hand, realize that if you have been with your partner through a long illness, a great deal of grieving has been done in advance. Then the death of a dear one can be almost a relief, and you may be ready for companionship, love, and sex much sooner than is conventionally thought to be proper.

This was true for **Stuart**. He had nursed his wife through seven long years of illness. Shortly after her death, he began to court **Donna**, and they married 10 months after his wife's death. This shocked some members of their conservative, religious community. But, according to Stuart, "I had a long, slow time to say goodbye to my wife. When God took her to Heaven, I knew He was right in taking her and that He has blessed my union with Donna."

WOMEN WHO LED SHELTERED LIVES

Women who have led sheltered lives in their marriages and are not ready to be out in the world alone may plunge into a relationship too soon after a death. Many older women come from a generation where they did not work, nor did they have experience in handling the finances of the home, much less the investments. Some seldom went any place without their husbands. For such women, being alone now can be quite frightening.

I was made aware of this some years ago when I led a small therapy group of widows, all quite advanced in years. Their husbands had handled all the family finances themselves. We spent time going over such practical matters as paying bills and balancing a checkbook. These women were apprehensive about going places alone. I gave homework assignments, and if a member succeeded in going for a cup of coffee alone, and later perhaps attending a movie by herself, she received applause and congratulations when she reported this achievement to the group.

Like the women in my group, it can be a challenge to learn new and more independent ways of functioning. Then an eventual new partnership could be a more equal one. However, many older women can be quite happy when a new partner takes care of many of their needs. They have lived long lives and need not be expected to change greatly.

MEN'S NEED FOR CLOSE TIES

Many men do not have close friends with whom they can intimately share their feelings. Their wives may have been their only close ties, and she may have been the one who arranged their social lives. Then when she dies, such a man can indeed feel lost. If he rushes into a relationship to fill that empty spot, it might work out if he finds the right woman. **David** and **Naomi** are an example of such a relationship working out well. David had a very close tie with his first wife. He had friendships with other men but as with many men, these friendships were based mainly on activities together, such as golfing and fishing. Usually these associations are not intimate, and as the men grow older, their activities and comradeships fade away, as they did in David's case. David rushed into a relationship with Naomi just a few months after his wife died. Fortunately, this marriage has lasted 13 years and has worked out well. David's wife now is his one really intimate friend and through her they have an active social life.

Often if a man chooses out of urgent need, he does not choose wisely. An alternative would be to take some time to learn to make close friendships on his own. Then he might be in a better position to enter into a relationship where a new partner is not his only source of emotional support. **John** is an example of such a man. He has a number of close men friends and does not depend solely on **Karin** for his social network.

HELP FOR THE BEREAVED AND DIVORCED

There are ways that both the bereaved and the divorced can find help. After a death, both men and women can obtain support through a grief group (usually found through a hospital or a hospice service) or by individual counseling. Grief groups deal not only with the initial grief but also with how to get on with your life alone and perhaps eventually to find a new partner. Groups for survivors of divorce are available through counseling agencies and private psychotherapists; sometimes they are advertised in local newspapers. Some divorce groups are self-led rather than being led by a professional.

Cliff was depressed after his divorce. In addition to reading extensively about relationships, he attended such a group. He reported, "I learned a great deal about myself, about my errors in choosing women, and about how I could be different the next time around. At times it was painful, but it was certainly worth the time and money."

After a divorce or a long, unsatisfactory union, many say they want a new relationship, but because of painful experiences they are distrustful. They may go through the first steps of searching but never find anyone who pleases them. On a deeper level, such an individual is not ready for commitment. This became clear to me when I was widowed. I joined an organization that helped people find new partners. After a while, I noticed that many of the same men, attractive and intelligent, remained in the organization for several years. I wondered why such individuals never found women who suited them.

Then Harold, a very handsome, intelligent, professional man, came to me for psychotherapy. Harold had a psychotic mother who had treated him cruelly as a child. He was then married for years to a very unstable woman, much like his mother. Harold's issue in coming to me was his desire to form a new relationship after his divorce. But inside he was terrified. He could not conceive of a woman who could be kind and loving. He was a man whom most women would like to be with, but he was afraid to become involved. After quite a few months of psychotherapy with me, Harold stopped longing to return to his very disturbed former wife. He began to take good care of himself and to look forward to new adventures. Perhaps now he might be ready to find an appropriate partner. He needed to take the first step of becoming happy inside himself before he was ready to start his search.

Harold provided my answer to the question of why those men remained for years on the organization's list for potential partners. On the mental level, they wanted to find someone, but on an emotional level, they were frightened. Many unsatisfactory relationships are a repetition of childhood trauma, as was Harold's. These painful experiences may then lead to an avoidance of commitment. Certainly there are many individuals who are perfectly content with being alone. It is the conflict between wanting intimacy and fear of it that provokes anxiety. If you, like Harold, fear a close relationship because of early pain, personal therapy might be appropriate.

If you are bereaved after a long marriage, you may need the developmental experiences of meeting other people. For both the widowed and the divorced, contacting interest groups like those listed in the next chapter, *Sources for a Search,* can be an appropriate first step. Such groups are helpful to those who are divorced, as through them individuals can meet and interact with members of the opposite sex who are kind and decent people and thus, become less gun-shy of forming new relationships. Young teenagers often form friendship groups of both sexes before dating, and surprisingly, the same principle may be true for you at this stage of your life.

Andy belonged to a singles group after his divorce, and the experience was an excellent transition period for him. Andy stated, "After a bad marriage and a difficult divorce, I went through some pretty hard times. It wasn't easy to trust women again. The singles groups were fun. I met a lot of nice women and began to realize that women are human beings too. It made me ready for **Joanne**."

THE BENEFITS OF INDEPENDENCE

Contrary to earlier psychological thinking, humans can continue to grow and develop as long as they live. **Karin** and **Naomi**, both widows after being in long marriages, gained self-confidence through employment and independent activities. The experiences of being independent and spreading their wings helped them to develop into more mature persons, and thus, made them ready for satisfying new relationships. I want to point out however, that there is no set standard for what is a "fully developed person." We each must decide this for ourselves.

IN SUMMATION

It is important to know yourself to be truly ready for a new relationship. Then you can be aware if you are becoming involved with an unsuitable partner merely to avoid being alone or to alleviate your grief. With self-knowledge, you prevent yourself from committing to an unsatisfactory relationship. If divorced, you may need help to resolve the internal conflict between the need for closeness and the fear of it.

Both the widowed and the divorced can benefit from involvement with various groups where they can meet others who have had similar experiences. Though it differs for each person, it takes time to be comfortable with your single self before you are ready to become part of a couple again.

Part of being ready is not only knowing yourself but also accepting yourself for who you are. I had difficulty doing this. After 35 years of a good marriage, with only one daughter and no grandchildren, I was lonely and longed for love and companionship. Yet I compared myself unfavorably with the many older single women I met who seemed perfectly content with their lot and with other widows who had no desire to find new partners. I thought I was somewhat deficient for wanting a man. I had to tell myself many times what I tell my clients: *to accept myself as I am.* I feel blessed to have found Jerry (he says he found me!). Without him I would have continued to be busy, and often happy, but with something very much missing.

Realize that feelings of loneliness are natural. Wanting someone to love and with whom to share your life is a normal and healthy desire. In the end, there is no set time after the dissolution of one relationship for the start of a new one. You, and you alone, can best judge when you are ready to start your search.

Chapter 23

SOURCES FOR A SEARCH

Once you are motivated and ready to find a companion, you should develop a plan of action. First, become aware of the people, places, and services that could lead you to potential contacts. In this chapter, we suggest some sources that can be found in many communities or through communications media like newspapers or the Internet. A good place to start is with your own network of acquaintances.

FRIENDS AND FORMER ACQUAINTANCES

Your friends want to see you fulfilled and happy. By describing your needs and interests to them, the potential is good for being introduced to someone whom you might find appealing. Another strategy is to attend high school or college reunions and perhaps, to look up former acquaintances or sweethearts who may now be widowed or divorced.

Leonard and **Barbara** worked in the same profession many years ago. They had developed a friendship and were attracted to each other but did not act upon it. Leonard was married, and Barbara was engaged at that time. After his wife's death, Leonard sought out Barbara. Their ease in being together and the chemistry between them had not changed. They are now in a successful marriage.

Be clear and specific with friends when indicating your interests and those desired in a potential partner (lifestyle, recreational pursuits, hobbies, religious preference, political views, and so forth).

See suggestions in Chapter 24 that can help you define desired traits in a partner.

My husband Jerry and I met through friends. He described to them what he wanted in a woman, and they contacted a friend of mine who thought I was a match. She called me, and I gave her permission to give Jerry my name, address, and phone number. And so it started.

With this approach you might "strike it right," although an obvious limitation to contacting friends or former acquaintances is that they may have no one to suggest, or their recommendation might not suit you. But it certainly can be worth the effort, and you might feel much safer with an acquaintance of a friend than with someone from more impersonal sources.

SENIOR CENTERS AND ACTIVITY GROUPS

Almost every community has a senior center that offers a variety of activities, some of which may be of interest to you. Often, involvement in a senior center leads to finding a group of compatible friends and possibly someone specific for you. But the hope of meeting that special person through a senior center may be limited, particularly for women, because of the paucity of single, available men. Also, women usually remain healthy longer than do men, so those men at the center who are available may not be as active or as vibrant as the women.

Many communities often organize social and recreational activities that are for seniors or that invite their participation. You can become involved in one or more activities that are enjoyable to you. These could possibly lead to meeting someone with similar interests. Service organizations such as the Kiwanis, Lions, and Rotarians, and recreational groups for card playing, hiking, bowling, dog training, and dancing are examples. Nature and environmental-interest groups, such as the Sierra Club and the Audubon Society may be helpful. Do you know of the Elderhostel organization for seniors (1-877-426-8056 and www.elderhostel.org) that sponsors numerous travel and educational activities? Watch for announcements of meetings and programs in newspapers, or inquire about them at a local senior or information center.

Whether or not you find a partner, you will be enriching your life by engaging in what really pleases you. If you do find someone who suits you, you will have similar interests to share in your relationship. **John** and **Karin** met while ballroom dancing, and they continued to very much enjoy dancing together. **Bill** and **Joyce** met when hiking with a club and now hike together regularly.

SINGLES GROUPS

Gatherings provide opportunities for divorced or widowed people to meet on a regular basis and to learn to know each other well. Such a group may be announced in the local newspaper or discovered through conversations with other people. Many interesting social and cultural activities can be enjoyed, even if you do not meet a special person. The disadvantage, again unhappily for women, is that often there are many more women than men in singles groups.

After some years of being widowed, I joined a singles group that was offered to graduates of the university that I had attended. It made my life much busier and more enjoyable. I attended parties, went to museums and concerts, and joined their book discussion group. As there were far more women than men in the group, I soon knew I would never meet a partner there, although I made quite a few new women friends.

On a more hopeful note, **Cliff**, after his divorce belonged to a singles group where he learned a great deal about women and relationships. Then, as a final bonus, he met his wife-to-be, **Janice**, at one of the group's dances. It might be easier for men to find partners, but both men and women certainly can enjoy the social advantages of a singles group.

CHURCH GROUPS

Churches and other religious organizations encourage members to participate in activities that can lead to forming friendships with those who have similar values. Church newsletters might contain personal ads that provide a means of meeting other individuals of the same faith. This is especially important if religion is central to your life. Faith was important to many of the couples interviewed. For **Naomi** and **David**, meeting at their temple was crucial to their forming a relationship. While **Donna** and **Stuart** did not meet in church, their seeing each other as good Christians made them acceptable partners to each other.

Becoming active in your church can enrich your life in many ways. It can be a source of emotional support and can offer you a chance to help others. If you meet that special person, you will be together in your beliefs and values.

PERSONAL ADS

Although some people feel awkward when placing or answering an advertisement, this is becoming an increasingly acceptable practice. Look through the personal columns in your local newspaper to see if a particular ad interests you. Or you might decide to place your own ad. Don't be discouraged if you do not see many senior entries. By frequently glancing through the personal page of your newspaper, you might find someone appropriate to contact and that someone may be awaiting your ad! **Ellen** and **Ralph** met this way.

For a newspaper announcement, you need to be brief and specific with a few lively words to describe yourself and the type of person you are seeking. The cost usually is minimal. To ensure privacy, an entry usually is given a mailbox address for writing or phoning. When you make a contact that seems appropriate, you should arrange to meet in a public place such as a coffee house. Be cautious until you feel safe and comfortable with the individual.

The chief disadvantage of this method is that you may meet some unacceptable individuals. By developing a good ear for phone conversations, you can weed some of them out immediately. If you meet a person who is unsuitable, make the meeting brief. Stay positive. With each encounter, you could have an interesting conversation and learn more about the opposite sex, even if that particular person is not someone you would want to see again. You can always end your time together with, "It was so nice meeting you—goodbye." Don't be afraid of hurting the other person's feelings. He or she has knowingly taken the same risk as you have. It is more cruel to promise another contact and then never follow through.

DATING SERVICES

Look for advertisements in the personal section of your local newspaper, or in publications of some religious organizations. Some of these services can be quite expensive, so inquire about fees, methods used to match people, and the potential for a person of your age and sex to find a partner.

Some dating services work on a direct, personal basis. You visit the service office, where you are interviewed to identify the qualities you desire in a partner. Then from their files, after reading personal descriptions and seeing photographs, you select one or more individuals to contact. Also, data about you can be added to their records for potentially interested clients to examine.

Be very cautious about investing a large sum of money in an expensive dating service. A friend of mine, an attractive woman in her early sixties, gave $2,000 to such a service. She believes it was one of the most foolish mistakes she's made in her life. The service had solicited her with a questionnaire that she completed and returned. Then they telephoned her many times, convincing her to go for an interview and to pay their fee. It was really a hard sell. They promised her 16 introductions, however she received only 7 recommendations, none of whom had the qualifications she so clearly outlined in her questionnaire and interview. She was so irate that she tried to sue the service, but they had already declared bankruptcy. If you decide to invest your hopes in an expensive dating service, I suggest that you ask for and carefully check references.

A happier story about a dating service relates to another friend of mine, also an attractive, interesting woman in her sixties. She joined a dating service for a minimal fee of $50 and then received a listing of men with brief descriptions of each one. She made selections that interested her and paid a small fee to receive a profile of each man and how to contact him. She was persistent for several years, meeting some interesting men, and now is living happily with the man of her choice. And she moved to another part of the country to be with him!

Because the pool of available men is smaller for older women, you might consider a dating service that draws from a large geographical area. First, however, you need to ask yourself if you would be willing to relocate if you found the right man. I believe the chances of men finding women they like from a dating service are greater, but still, be careful to investigate the service you choose.

THE INTERNET

Computer training is available in many senior centers and local education programs. The Internet provides many opportunities to find information about dating services, and e-mail allows you to communicate with a person who may seem interesting. If you are not computer literate, ask a friend or even a grandchild for guidance.

By browsing with Netscape or Microsoft Internet Explorer software, or by using a search engine such as Yahoo (www.yahoo.com) or AltaVista (www.altavista.com), you can find home pages for dating websites. At the time of this writing, there are personals.yahoo.com (for adults of all ages), thirdage.com (for those who are 45–64), and www.seniornet.com (65 and older). Also in this last category are www.seniorwomen.com and www.seniormen.com. Calling up a bulletin board service such as Usenet News permits you to post and respond to messages, while chat groups such as www.match.com and www.mplayer.com will allow you to communicate with others of similar age and interests.

Be careful when using the Internet not to exchange vital information such as your address or phone number, and do not make commitments until you have the opportunity to meet face-to-face in a public place and feel comfortable with the individual. The advice about phone calls and personal meetings under *Personal Ads* applies also to the Internet. Remember that someone can write wonderfully on e-mail but not be the same at all in a personal encounter. But who knows!

Evaluate the practicality of the sources available to you and the ones you believe will be the most useful. Then utilize the planning suggestions given in the next chapter to examine your own values and your expectations of a potential partner.

Chapter 24

EXAMINING WHAT YOU WANT IN A PARTNER

After establishing your desire and readiness to find a companion, and being prepared to approach sources, you should ask yourself the following questions.

- What is most important to me in life?
- What are my values, and what lifestyle do I want to share with someone?
- What characteristics would I like in a partner?

The answers to these questions will form a framework to help you define your own values and the type of person you hope to find. When you do meet someone, discuss together your common interests and aspirations. The following are matters for you to consider before you start your search and as you become acquainted with potential partners. Some items might not be appropriate for when you first meet but can be explored as your relationship develops.

WHAT IS YOUR PHILOSOPHY OF LIFE AND YOUR VALUE SYSTEM?

By reading the interview chapters of this book, you will find many persons expressing the beliefs and values important to them, and how their partners share or understand and respect their views. It is not necessary for a partner to share all your views but respect for differences is important. Often over time, by listening to each other, the differences in viewpoints are reduced.

Janice, when she first met **Cliff**, was positively impressed because they shared the same values about social issues. She, as a child psychologist, and he, as a health-care provider, were concerned about the care of children and wanted help for families living in poverty.

Another positive fit in values was found by **Donna** and **Stuart**. Donna saw Stuart as a good, moral, upright Christian man who did not smoke or drink. They were both very devout Christians, and Donna joined Stuart's church.

Edna and **Seymour** are an example of a couple having different belief systems who were able to comfortably accept each other's differences. Edna believes in reincarnation and the importance of astrological signs. Seymour does not hold these beliefs but is able to give Edna the respect of not trying to change her convictions. To Seymour, Judaism is very important. Edna has not converted to his faith but is active with him in temple activities.

Gayle, in describing what she wanted in a partner, was very articulate in a prayer to her goddess: "a man who is open-minded, comfortable with my feminism and my beliefs in a different theological system than most people have. He doesn't have to believe as I do but be comfortable with my believing my way." To Gayle, **Jim** fit this description.

WHAT PHYSICAL FEATURES DO YOU FIND DESIRABLE IN A PARTNER?

Physical features are often the first characteristic noticed. **Andy** was caught by **Joanne's** walk, which he said "had a lively bounce." **David** liked **Naomi's** well-built body and her artistic manner of dressing. In turn, Naomi thought David "looked adorable in shorts." **Mary** noticed that **Fred** was handsome and well dressed. **Ed** saw **Laura** as beautiful and loved her smile. All the interviewees found other features of their partners, beyond physical ones, that were important to them as their relationship developed.

Certainly you should consider what physical traits you find desirable, but making them the prime factor is a narrow and confining way of looking for a partner. When I met Jerry, I was neither impressed nor repelled by his looks. My friend who called me about him had inquired as to his appearance and told me he was "just so-so." Now that I've come to love him, I find him extremely attractive.

As you come to care for your partner, a greater physical attraction can develop. Remember, as we age, our appearances change. A number of the couples I interviewed showed me photos of themselves when they first met or were married. Some of them were smashingly good looking but are no longer as attractive. Yet, they still love each other and find their mates physically appealing.

HOW DO YOU BOTH MATCH UP INTELLECTUALLY AND SOCIALLY?

When you first meet someone, it is not too difficult to know if that person is intellectually stimulating. Does he or she hold your interest when you talk, or do you find your mind wandering? Does he or she talk *too* much, particularly about him or herself? The ability to listen to another person is important. And remember that the person you find intellectually stimulating may not necessarily have the same level of education as you do. **Barbara** says of **Leonard**, "He is less educated but more intelligent than any of my previous husbands."

A wide variety of experiences can make a prospective partner interesting to you. **Stuart** had traveled extensively and lived in many countries. This was fascinating to **Donna**.

One couple clearly stated what attracted them each to the other. Says **Gayle** of **Jim**, "He's very interesting to talk with. He has eclectic interests in many subjects, and he is very perceptive." And Jim says of Gayle, "It's fascinating to listen to her talk."

Consider how well the other person interacts with your family and friends. These aspects of social behaviors are important in any developing relationship. **Gayle**, after meeting **Jim**, was pleased with how he interacted with her friends at a dinner gathering. In another situation, shortly after they met, **Ellen** took **Ralph** to visit her friends. If he had not fit in well, Ellen doubts if their relationship would have continued.

I had known Jerry only about a month when I invited him to join me in visiting some very good friends. They liked him tremendously, and we all got along very well. This was very important to me and was a strong factor in my realizing how much I cared for him.

Intellectual and social compatibility are qualities that will remain important to a couple throughout life, so consider them carefully. These traits may well add variety and zest to a relationship.

WHAT HOUSING ARRANGEMENTS WOULD YOU BOTH PREFER?

Consider your preferred living style—city house, apartment, or condominium; rural or waterfront location; retirement community;

or even major time spent traveling in a motor home. Usually a discussion of these preferences will occur further along in your relationship, when you are considering living together or marrying. An exception is **Ellen,** who in her newspaper ad specifically stated that she wanted a man who likes recreational-vehicle living. She and **Ralph** are now living and traveling in their motor home.

Of course, once you are involved, you will know where your partner lives and how attached he or she is to a residence. As your time together increases, it is usual to spend more time at one partner's home. This may be because it is larger, more comfortable, or more conveniently located.

This brings up the question of where to live once you marry or decide to live together. A number of the men interviewed were quite content to move into their partners' homes. **Leonard**, **Paul**, **Bill**, and **Jim** left their city or suburban homes to happily reside in their partners' country residences. The change for these men gave them new interests and activities in their retirement. **Paul**, who was raised on a farm, thought **Ruth's** home was familiar and comfortable, yet he kept his large, suburban home for five years, which was located at a distance. Paul and Ruth visited there frequently. He finally sold it because after five years he was ready to say goodbye to the home in which he had raised his family.

Ed relocated to **Laura's** home because his house held such sad memories of his wife's death. **Mary** moved into **Fred's** larger and more elegant house after their marriage, although it was in an entirely different community, away from her family and friends. The transition was difficult for her, and they eventually moved back to her community, buying an apartment together in a retirement development. Similarly, **Edna** and **Seymour** started out in her home but eventually bought into a retirement community together. **Naomi** and **David** did the same.

Often a couple initially lives in one of their homes, but eventually they buy a new residence together. This can give a real sense of it now becoming *their* home. Also, as we age, retirement communities offer real advantages. (This topic is considered in Chapter 26.)

Then there are those who choose to live separately, as do **Nancy** and **Pat**, and **Carol** and **Ron**. The partners in each couple have the advantage of living close to each other, making it easy to have both separate and together time and space.

Jerry and I had no such advantage. I lived in a medium-size city and he in the country, more than three hours' driving distance away. For the first nine months, we commuted back and forth. Mostly I visited him, spending a week at a time at his house. Because the distance was too great and we wanted to be together, after nine months I moved into Jerry's home. Before I met Jerry, I never dreamed I would leave the community where I had lived for more than 35 years. Jerry couldn't accept city living, so I knew it was I who would move. It helped me to have the attitude that the move would be a new adventure for me.

I am still in transition. At first I returned to my city home twice a month to meet with clients, then once a month, and now only once every few months. My practice has transferred entirely to this rural community. My daughter now lives in my city home, so I can return there occasionally to visit friends and to enjoy restaurants, shopping, and cultural activities the city has to offer. Periodically, Jerry spends short periods of time with me there.

HOW IMPORTANT TO EACH OF YOU IS YOUR PARTNER'S FINANCIAL SITUATION AND SHARING OF EXPENSES?

As with housing preferences, finances might not be discussed until later in your relationship but it should not be too difficult to ascertain an individual's financial situation early. You need to ask yourself, "How important is this issue?" Here is how some couples handle their finances.

Karin, **Gayle**, and **Joanne** are all with men less financially well off than themselves and have no problem with it. When Karin and **John** travel, they do so at modest expense. Gayle pays **Jim's** travel expenses.

Paul is much more comfortable financially than is **Ruth** and pays for their trips, as traveling is especially important to him. Because he is less careful with money and makes many long-distance telephone calls, Ruth was somewhat annoyed. Paul now pays for these calls, solving that problem.

Before you actually live together or marry, it is important to discuss how expenses will be shared for the household, entertainment, and travel. More details of how the couples handle financial matters are described in Chapter 21. Also consider any need for a pre-marital agreement, wills, trusts, and other financial or legal matters. (See Chapter 26 for information about these subjects.)

WHAT ATTITUDES DO YOU BOTH HAVE REGARDING EACH OTHER'S CHILDREN AND GRANDCHILDREN?

Getting along with each other's children, and their acceptance of you, are important in a successful relationship. To what degree would children accept a new partner? What are some ways to encourage and support positive interactions fairly early in your developing relationship? And how might you handle resentments or negative attitudes?

We treat this topic in Chapter 16, giving many examples from the couples interviewed. Often, after an initial shock, children frequently accept and support a parent's new arrangement. But whatever your children's reactions, your relationship with your partner should be your first consideration.

HOW DO YOU EACH REACT TO AGE DIFFERENCES AND HEALTH CONDITIONS?

While you may meet someone close to your present age, there is also the likelihood that you might be attracted to someone of an appreciably different age—older or younger. Realize that in a reasonable length of time, health problems and other symptoms of aging can become evident and must be prepared for and accepted. As you read the interviews, you will find many situations of wide age differences (10 years or more) and even the beginnings of necessary caretaking by one partner for the other.

With **Naomi** and **David**, and **Laura** and **Ed**, the women have begun to assume the role of caretakers for older men. Though **David** is only three years older than **Naomi**, his health and memory have begun to deteriorate. Naomi is a very active person and is open about her unhappiness with having to give up many of her interests to stay home with David. This unhappiness does not interfere with her love and concern for her husband. The reader needs to know that feelings of unhappiness about caretaking do not mean you love your partner less or that you do not do what is necessary. Groups are available that can provide encouragement and support for caretakers.

Laura is age 80, while **Ed** is 90. He has had many serious operations, but in this case, Laura is more accepting of the caretaker role than is Naomi. You need to ask yourself, "Do I love this person enough to stand by him (or her) and, if it becomes necessary, to care for him (or her) until the end?"

In time, share information with each other about present health conditions and support that may eventually be necessary. Discuss the advisability of both of you taking blood tests for AIDS before becoming sexually involved. As of 1999 about 78,000 people, 50 and older, had developed AIDS, up from 17,000 a decade ago.

(Reported by the Center for Disease Control and Prevention, May 2000.)

People of even the same age vary greatly in physical vitality and intellectual alertness. Therefore, look beyond age differences. **Gayle**, 10 years older than **Jim**, is an extremely active and vibrant person who, when asked about their age differences, said with a smile, "Yes, Jim's younger than I am, and therefore it's more difficult for him too keep up with me—right?"

Jerry is nine years older than I am, but walks so fast that I almost need to run to keep up with him. And you should see him climbing a ladder and trees in our orchard!

WHAT ARE EACH OF YOUR FOOD PREFERENCES AND NUTRITIONAL HABITS?

This matter can become an important factor within a relationship and can either lead to satisfaction and support or to conflict and disagreements. As a relationship develops, nutritional likes and dislikes and the need for special diets become evident. Accepting change to reach a middle ground and exploring new ideas, all need open-minded considerations.

Carol and **Ron** became more and more aware of alternative nutritional practices and together, changed their eating habits. Now both are practicing vegetarians and participate in programs that encourage this style of eating.

WHAT ARE EACH OF YOUR INTERESTS FOR RECREATIONAL ACTIVITIES?

Sharing activities such as exercise and sports, entertainment, travel, and hobbies can contribute to the development of a stronger relationship. Sometimes one partner is already involved in sports such as golf or tennis, and the other learns to play in order to enjoy time together. If you met through an interest group, it is natural to continue this activity as a couple. Anne, a 66-year-old widowed client of mine, met her husband-to-be while bird watching, and as she told me, "We now love to travel together on birding trips."

A central theme of this book is the balance between separateness and togetherness. Certainly it is a plus to have mutual interests, but a couple often needs time apart, especially during the retirement years, when work and children no longer provide separateness. Most of our couples have arranged their lives so they have both separate and together times. **Edna** and **Seymour** are good examples of this balance. They play bridge and golf together and volunteer at a shelter for the homeless. By herself, Edna is a potter and a gardener. Seymour, on his own, collects Indian arrowheads and plays a leadership role in his religious organization.

DO YOU ACCEPT EACH OTHER'S PROFESSIONAL, BUSINESS, OR VOLUNTEER ACTIVITIES?

Participating in ongoing and new enterprises offer both financial and intellectual benefits. You must decide whether to encourage and support such efforts by your partner. Often older people, wishing to remain active, serve as volunteers in the community. As long as such work does not excessively drain one's energy or detract from personal or family affairs, the participant can greatly benefit.

Volunteer or professional activities can help the balance of separateness and togetherness. In their small apartment in a retirement home, **Laura** and **Ed** are very much together, but Laura, age 80, finds time alone by doing volunteer work as a tutor in a nearby elementary school. **Janice** practices part-time as a psychologist, while her husband **Cliff** volunteers in organizations serving their community. **Gayle** is active in many community organizations in addition to her work as a sculptor and a proprietor of an art gallery, while **Jim** receives income as a freelance editor. They work together on Gayle's projects, with both providing ideas and Jim doing the final editing and computer work.

When you begin to be involved with someone, consider how that person reacts to your activities if you still work even part-time or serve as a volunteer. How do you respond to your partner's employment or volunteer service? Jealousy of the time spent in these involvements may indicate an insecure person and trouble ahead.

CAN YOU ACCEPT YOUR PARTNER'S FRIENDSHIP WITH A FORMER SPOUSE?

Because most older couples have adult children, they often do not have the frequent contact with a former spouse, as when younger children are involved. However there might still be a platonic friendship between your partner and a former wife or husband. Could you accept this without undue jealousy? **John** is still quite friendly with his former wife, the mother of his children, from whom he's been divorced for many years. **Karin**, who lives separately from John, accepts this friendship.

WHAT INTEREST DO YOU BOTH HAVE FOR KEEPING A PET?

Possibly one or both of you already have a dog or cat. We know that an animal can be an important part of any household, but some people do not like the responsibility of the care involved, or they may be allergic to animals. On the other hand, there are pleasures in having an animal and health benefits can result from reacting to an animal's antics and companionship. Realize however, that arrangements for boarding are necessary when you are away from home for any length of time. **Joyce** has a cat, and **Bill** has brought his dog into her home. **Leonard** went to **Barbara's** home with a dog that happily plays with her dog and cat. **Stuart** objected to **Donna's** many pets. To compromise, she kept only one cat, that Stuart learned to accept. When forming a new relationship be clear with each other as to what is acceptable to each of you in terms of pets.

A TIME FOR ACTION

Once you are clear in your mind about the type of person you desire, it may be time to take action. If you find someone of interest through a church or an activity group, you will have had a chance to get to know that person in a social context. When you are ready, you might ask him or her to join you for coffee, dinner, a movie, or whatever you both fancy.

If you have located a person whom you have not yet met, an initial contact may be made by mail, e-mail, or telephone. A letter should be general and not lengthy (two pages maximum) yet provide sufficient information about yourself to stimulate the other individual to respond. As an example, see the letter below that Jerry wrote to Edith.

> Dear Edith,
>
> I recently visited a friend and his wife, Bill and Joan Jackson, whom I have not seen for some time. During our conversation I told him that my wife had passed away two years ago and that I was interested in sharing my life now with someone who has similar interests and has both emotional and intellectual needs that match mine. Last Friday I received a phone call from Bill to tell me that his wife, Joan, had spoken to a friend, Lynn Martin, and your name was mentioned as someone who

might be interested in meeting me. I decided to write you this letter as an introduction and then follow up with a phone call. You are welcome to give me a call when you receive this letter.

I am in my mid-70s, 5'9" tall, slender, and in good physical condition. I act much younger than my age, both physically and mentally. I had a grandmother who attained 103 years, and my mother was 98 at her passing, so I have the right genes!

I find hiking, swimming, and other outdoor activities to my liking. For the mind, I am a retired university professor and author of three textbooks. I continue to write and engage in some professional consultations. I am interested in good nutritional practices, listening to Big Bands and Broadway show music, national and world events, wholesome television entertainment, and have the desire to do some traveling with a companion.

I left my city residence earlier this year and have settled in a comfortable home in the peaceful, slow-going foothills. Although I like to visit the "big city" periodically, I prefer to live in this natural, non-stressful environment. Twice a week I join a seniors' hiking group, and we explore wonderful places in the mountains and elsewhere. You should see the waterfalls this year!

I would like to share my interests with a lady who is happy in jeans, likes to grow and pick her own fresh vegetables and fruits, but periodically would dress up to spend time together in other activities.

Let's make contact and go from there. I'll wait a few days until I am sure you have received this letter.

Looking forward,
Jerry Kemp

A phone call, either as an initial contact or after your letter or e-mail, can give you a more personal sense of your possible partner. The voice and manner of speaking tell so much. Then, if you are still interested, you can suggest a brief meeting in person in a safe, public place. An hour together can give you a feeling for the person and how well you both match up. The time can be extended if the two of you are really hitting it off.

Develop a plan of action! You need to have a vision of how best to move toward your goal … *and good luck!*

Less than a month after first meeting, Edith wrote this poem for Jerry:

Jerry, Jerry, I'm so merry
That I've met you.
How could anyone who knows you
Ere forget you.
Time will tell what comes of us,
But for now it's marvelous.

Section Four

USEFUL INFORMATION FOR OLDER COUPLES

This Section consists of practical treatment of important topics that all older individuals and couples need to consider.

A number of useful references for further, more detailed information are cited at the end of each chapter.

Chapter 25

HEALTHY LIFESTYLE FOR LONGEVITY AND HAPPINESS

We continue to hear a great deal about the many factors that can contribute to good health and a long life, but much information and many recommendations often contradict past findings, leaving a person confused. This may be due to newspaper and other media reporters highlighting unusual findings to attract attention. Yet there are many sound principles and practices proven to contribute to a healthy lifestyle. You're never too old to take advantage of this information, especially if you can be helped to recognize the benefits to your body. Please read ahead. You might be positively reinforced for the good things you already do, or be motivated to take actions that could be beneficial to you. Isn't it worthwhile to try to live a few extra healthy, enjoyable years?

To help you do this, after reading the chapter, judge your own practices and consider changes you might make in your lifestyle by answering the questions we pose at the end. For more detailed information about most topics, see the list of useful references at the conclusion of the chapter.

PHYSICAL EXERCISE

There is unanimous agreement that exercise is the single most important anti-aging measure anyone can follow, regardless of age, disability, or general level of fitness. A sedentary lifestyle accelerates nearly every unwanted aspect of aging. Among other benefits, physical activity slows the erosion of muscle strength, improves body balance and flexibility, and maintains better cardiovascular and respiratory functions. It also helps with weight control, thus limiting the risk of developing diabetes; it contributes to improved cholesterol level profiles and increases bone mass, helping to prevent osteoporosis. Exercise also facilitates digestion, promotes efficient bowel function, and reduces insomnia. It can improve one's outlook on life, preventing or alleviating depression by producing endorphins (chemicals released by the body which have been linked to an elevation of mood); and by pumping blood to the brain, it helps a person think more clearly. The merits of physical activity are equally beneficial for women as they are for men.

To be effective, an exercise routine should include three major components of fitness. Modify this advice by considering the condition of your own health.

Endurance Activities

These include any type of total body movement that increases the demand placed on the cardiovascular and respiratory systems. The most popular are brisk walking, hiking, jogging, low-impact aerobics, swimming, using a treadmill or other machines, bicycling, and golfing without using a cart. A minimum of 30–45 minutes of activity, at least four times a week, with a gradual increase in extent and number of sessions, can positively affect blood pressure and other bodily functions. Gradually push yourself to cause some shortness of breath that raises your pulse rate and even sweat a little. These responses are indicators of positive benefits to your body.

If walking is your main activity, do not stroll. Try to include some uphill routes to put extra pressure on your system. On the level, try to work your pace up to 2½ to 3 miles an hour for best benefit. And when entering a multi-story building, instead of taking the elevator or escalator to the second floor, climb the stairs. Wear comfortable walking shoes that do not slip at the heel or pinch at the toes. For fun and motivation, obtain and wear a pedometer that can count steps, distance walked, and even calories burned. Twelve thousand or more steps a day can indicate that you have walked enough to benefit your health.

Strength Activities

Lifting weights not only builds muscles, but makes joints stronger and more supple, and will slow or even reverse many age-related problems including fatigue and walking difficulty. For postmenopausal women, who lose bone as hormone levels decline, strength activities can build bone density. Use light weights (1 to 10 pounds) to engage arm and chest muscles in resistance exercises. Do sit-ups or chin-ups to work the major muscle groups. Build up gradually to 12 repetitions of three different muscular activities for three sessions a week. As your muscles comfortably handle the exercise, gradually increase size of weights for use in resistance exercises.

Water aerobics, offered by many facilities that have swimming pools, is a gentle way of strengthening muscles through body movements against the force of water and is therapeutic to the joints. Because of the buoyancy of water, this method of exercise is particularly appropriate for individuals who find it difficult to participate in other forms of exercise.

Stretching

Stretching should be an important part of any exercise routine. It improves flexibility and balance, allowing you to move your joints through their full range of motion, while easing muscle soreness. Extend each part of your body—arms, legs, feet, back, and neck—until you feel some resistance without pain. Hold each stretch for 15–30 seconds. Relax and repeat several times. Stretch at the beginning of an exercise when your muscles have begun to warm up and then again when cooling down after a workout. (For more detailed information and illustrations, refer to the free publication, *Exercise: A Guide from the National Institute on Aging*, in the references on page 317.)

For some people, learning yoga and Chinese tai chi, which are partially stretching exercises, can be beneficial and pleasurable. Tai chi involves many dance-like postures performed in slow-motion sequences. It calls for concentration, controlled breathing, and balanced shifting of body weigh. It is an invaluable aid in improving an older individual's balance, for whom falls can be disabling. Many senior centers offer yoga, tai chi, and easy, low-impact exercise classes.

Make exercise a part of daily life. Choose one or more activities that are appropriate and enjoyable for you. Consider activities such as tennis and golf for general exercising. How much you can and should do depends on your general health, present level of fitness, and any degree of disability. Finally, consider these important practices and precautions:

- Talk with your doctor before starting an exercise program.
- Listen to your body. Be alert to dizziness, nausea, breathlessness, or chest pain that could indicate a level of distress.

- Try to exercise with a partner or participate in group sessions at a senior center or elsewhere—it's good motivation and offers some competition.

- Drink water before, during, and after exercising.

- Exercising too hard provides less benefit than a steady, low-impact program.

- Establish a habit so that exercise becomes an integral part of your daily routine.

A HEALTHY DIET

Often we hear or read about what a specific food product can do for health. For example, unsaturated oil, fresh fish, and wine are reported to prevent heart disease; broccoli, tomatoes, green tea, and soy foods can prevent cancer; and so forth. While the specific benefits promoted may be more than research has established, there are sensible reasons to emphasize certain groups of foods and reduce others in your diet. A properly balanced daily diet should include the following (sizes of servings and some suggested foods are indicated in parentheses):

- **Water**: eight 8-ounce glasses

- **Grains and bread**: 6–11 servings (1–2 slices of whole-grain bread; one-half cup of cooked brown rice or whole-grain pasta; one cup of non-sugared breakfast cereal; one-half cup of whole-grain cooked cereal)

- **Vegetables**: 3–5 servings (one-half cup, raw or cooked; one cup of a leafy vegetable such as spinach; three-quarters cup of juice)

- **Fruits**: 2–4 servings (one-half cup fresh; one-quarter cup dried; a melon wedge; half a grapefruit; one apple, one orange; three-quarters cup of a juice)

- **Protein-rich**: 2–3 servings (5–7 ounces of lean meat, fish, or skinless poultry; one-half cup of beans, pasta, or a soy product; one-third cup of nuts)

- **Dairy products**: 2–3 low-fat servings (one cup of milk; 8 ounces of yogurt; one-half cup of cottage cheese; 1½ ounces of cheese)

- **Sweets, fats, and oils**: sparing use (olives; avocado; walnuts or almonds; canola, sunflower, or olive oil)

- **Salt intake**: less than 2,400 mg, or about one teaspoon total in all foods, including what is indicated on processed packaged foods

See the diagram of the recommended *USDA Daily Food Guide Pyramid* in the *Self-Evaluation Exercise* on page 313. A daily diet containing the specified food groups in the amounts indicated can cut the risk of heart disease, colon cancer, and diabetes, while decreasing common gastrointestinal problems and constipation. Switching from a high-fat to a low-fat diet often reduces total cholesterol and can produce small declines in blood pressure.

For an assessment of your present diet, visit the USDA's online *Interactive Healthy Eating Index* at www.usda.gov.cnpp. You report the types and quantities of the foods you eat each day, obtaining a score on the quality of your daily diet as compared to the Food Guide Pyramid.

Also, watch the increasing publicity being given to Mediterranean-type diets which substantial research is proving to have worthwhile benefits. For example: There is a 50 percent to 70 percent lower risk of repeated heart attacks with this diet, compared to conventional Western diets (reported in the *Environmental Nutrition* newsletter, March 1999).

Develop the habit of reading the contents and tabulations of nutritional facts (serving size, calories, fat content, cholesterol, sodium, carbohydrates, and proteins) on packaged food labels. Make choices based on your dietary needs in terms of this information. Following is a listing of proportional components for a healthful diet, as reported in the *Harvard Men's Health Watch* newsletter (March 1999).

Food or Nutrient	Healthful Standard (daily)
Cholesterol	Less than 300 mg
Saturated fat	Less than 10% of calories
Polyunsaturated fat	3–7% of calories
Dietary fiber	27–40 grams
Simple carbohydrates	Less than 10% of calories
Complex carbohydrates	50–70% of calories
Protein	10–15% of calories
Fruits and vegetables	More than 400 grams
Nuts and seeds	More than 30 grams

Meanings of food terms used in this table are:

- *Saturated fats* are usually solid at room temperature and come from animal sources—butter, milk fat, meat fat, and two vegetable oils (coconut and palm). Margarines and shortenings are similar to saturated fats.

- *Polyunsaturated fats* are usually liquid at room temperature and come from plants and fish—corn, safflower, and sesame oils are varieties, while olive, peanut, canola, and avocado are the preferable *monounsaturated* oils.

- *Simple carbohydrates* are the sugars derived from fruits and vegetables—table sugar, glucose, fructose, lactose in milk.

- *Complex carbohydrates* consist primarily of starches, wheat, grains, and other fiber products that occur in plant foods.

Although it may be difficult to relate milligrams (mg), grams, and percentages to actual amounts of foods consumed during a day, the above table can give some indication of relative amounts in food categories that comprise an acceptable diet.

If you are overweight, develop a program of regular exercise to burn calories, select a healthy diet as described above, while reducing refined and junk foods containing high amounts of sugar and white flour (often listed first or second in quantity on nutritional labels).

DIETARY SUPPLEMENTS

While a sound diet theoretically can provide all the vitamins and minerals you need, many older adults show deficiency in vitamins B6, B12, D, and E; in addition, folic acid and calcium. A standard senior-formulated multivitamin can fill most of these gaps. Often, both men and women need additional calcium and Vitamins C, B12, and E which limit the harmful effects of oxygen free-radicals (cellular waste products that have been associated with aging and many age-related illnesses) and may improve the body's immune system.

Many multivitamin/multimineral supplements are available on the market that contain varying ingredients and strengths. What should be included in such a product and with what strength? On page 302 are recommendations from *Environmental Nutrition*, August 1998, derived from standards set by the National Academy of Sciences and the Council for Responsible Nutrition. (Abbreviations: IU—International Unit, mg—milligram, mcg—microgram, n/a—not available.)

Older people tend to eat less, yet they need more of several nutrients than do younger people. Items in the left column, marked with a *, may require the higher standard, as listed in the "Not to Exceed per Day" column. Check the dietary supplements you are taking (or should be taking), and see how the ingredients compare with the recognized amounts in this table.

ALCOHOL CONSUMPTION

Moderate consumption of alcohol is acceptable and may even provide some cardiovascular benefit. For someone who does not drink alcohol, the juice of red or purple grapes may have some of the same cardiovascular benefits as does wine. At present there are no conclusive indications of this benefit.

The Department of Agriculture defines moderate consumption as no more than one 5-ounce glass of wine (equivalent to 12 ounces of beer or 1.5 ounces of 80-proof distilled spirits) daily for women and no more than twice as much for men. However, some medical conditions and medications require abstinence from alcohol.

Nutrient	Amount per Tablet	% Daily Value	Not to Exceed per Day
Vitamin A	5,000 IU	100%	10,000 IU
Vitamin C	60 mg	100%	1,000 mg
Vitamin D*	400 IU	100%	800 IU
Vitamin E*	30 IU	100%	1,200 IU
Thiamin (B1)	1.5 mg	100%	n/a
Riboflavin (B2)	1.7 mg	100%	n/a
Niacinamide (B3)	20 mg	100%	35 mg
Vitamin B6	2 mg	100%	100 mg
Folic Acid	400 mcg	100%	1,000 mcg
Vitamin B12	6 mcg	100%	n/a
Biotin	30 mcg	10%	n/a
Pantothenic Acid	10 mg	100%	n/a
Calcium*	200 mg	20%	2,500 mg
Iron*	18 mg	100%	65 mg
Phosphorus	10 mg	1%	4,000 mg
Iodine	150 mcg	100%	1,000 mcg
Magnesium	100 mg	25%	350 mg
Zinc	15 mg	100%	30 mg
Copper	2 mg	100%	9 mg
Potassium	35 mg	1%	n/a
Vitamin K	40 mcg	50%	n/a
Selenium	35 mcg	50%	200 mcg
Manganese	2 mg	100%	10 mg
Chromium	25 mcg	21%	1,000 mcg
Molybdenum	25 mcg	33%	350 mcg
Chlorine	340 mg	10%	n/a
Nickel	5 mcg	none	n/a
Silicon	2 mg	none	n/a
Vanadium	10 mcg	none	n/a
Boron	150 mcg	none	n/a
Tin	10 mcg	none	n/a

Aging increases alcohol sensitivity primarily because older body tissues hold less water than do younger tissues. Consequentially, a given amount of alcohol is more potent to an older adult than to a younger person of comparable height and weight. The result is a greater potential for intoxication, drug interactions, and side effects after fewer drinks. The older you are, the more cautious you should be about drinking anything other than in small amounts.

Women are more sensitive to alcohol than men because they produce less of the enzyme that breaks down alcohol. Studies show that the average woman achieves a higher blood-alcohol level and becomes as intoxicated after drinking half the amount of alcohol consumed by the average man. Smaller body size also can increase alcohol's potency because less body water is available to dilute the alcohol.

For older people, factors such as retirement, failing health, grief, loneliness, or living on a limited income can trigger excessive alcohol use. At first, the tendency is to use alcohol as a relief or an escape, but a dependency can become dangerous. Excessive alcohol use can lead to addiction and consequent liver damage. It is important for family and friends to be alert to subtle changes in an individual's behavior that could signal a developing problem with alcohol.

DAILY WATER INTAKE

Virtually all chemical processes in the body either take place in water or require it. Adequate hydration is important for optimal organ functions. Water also helps maintain body temperature and keeps internal membranes moist so that oxygen and other gasses can be exchanged. Older adults are vulnerable to dehydration, especially in warm weather. In addition to ingesting the water content of fruits and vegetables, drink eight glasses of pure water or other water-based fluids a day. Also remember to drink water while exercising, especially if you perspire.

SMOKING

Serious illness can result from smoking cigarettes and cigars. The cancer-causing substances in smoke, called carcinogens, are absorbed into the blood, which carries them to parts of the body that they can harm. A pack-a-day smoker is four times more likely to develop congestive heart failure and lung cancer than is a non-smoker. There is clear evidence that when someone stops smoking, about five years later, the person has reduced the risk for developing heart disease to the same degree as someone who has never smoked. It may however, take up to 15 years for the risk of lung cancer to return to the level of a nonsmoker. Quitting also decreases the risk of stroke, some other cancers, chronic bronchitis, and emphysema. It may also improve the cosmetic appearance of the skin and increase circulation. As the saying goes, "it's never too late to quit … the benefits are there."

EXPOSURE TO THE SUN

Aging skin and eyes are vulnerable to sun damage because protective pigment diminishes over time, permitting greater penetration of harmful rays. Although a small amount of sunlight is needed to produce vitamin D, too much exposure increases the risk of skin cancer. Ultraviolet damage is cumulative and may take years to show up. In addition, the sun can cause significant cosmetic damage. Most skin wrinkles, discoloration, and texture changes are directly related to sunlight. For protection use a sunscreen with a sun protection factor (SPF) of 15 or higher, wear a wide-brimmed hat, and use protective clothing over your entire body, including your arms. Finally, be sure to wear good-quality sunglasses outdoors to filter out ultraviolet rays that affect the eyes.

SEXUAL ACTIVITY

Continuing an active and enjoyable sex life adds immeasurably to physical and mental health. As with exercise, it increases endorphins that make you feel better all day. (Most older folks interviewed for this book engage in sexual activity in the morning.) If you don't have a partner, and if it doesn't clash with your religious or moral convictions, masturbation can be an acceptable sexual activity for single adults.

Regular exercise, a good diet, and avoiding tobacco and excess alcohol, all help to reduce the risk of developing chronic diseases. This limits the need to take medications that impair sexual functioning. Refer to Chapter 17, *Health and Sexuality,* to learn about the sex life of the older couples interviewed. Their experiences could surprise you!

When considering sexual activity, an alert needs to be sounded. There is evidence that seniors comprise one of the fastest-growing HIV/AIDS-infected populations. At one time, blood transmissions were considered to be the source of this problem. Today, with many divorced and widowed older adults being sexually active, it is more likely that unprotected sexual contact is the likely cause. There is also a good possibility that AIDS may go undiagnosed. Not only are many elderly people reluctant to discuss their intimate behaviors with their doctors, but the symptoms can conflict with common effects of old age—weight loss, depression, and mental impairment. Recognize the dangers of unsafe sex.

REDUCING STRESS

Studies show that anger, stress, and anxiety impair the immune system. These factors can increase the risk of heart disease, stroke, and susceptibility to other illness. During a stressful situation, the body's adrenal glands release adrenaline, which raises the heart rate and blood pressure, increasing the heart's workload and magnifying its need for oxygen. Stress also can cause spasms that narrow the arteries and activate blood platelets that initiate the clotting process in these arteries, thus triggering heart attacks.

It is important to structure your life to reduce negative feelings. Identify the situations that bother you most and try to change them. Learn to recognize the signs of building tensions such as a racing pulse, fast breathing, tight stomach, or a jumpy, restless feeling. When you recognize these signals, take steps to relieve the tension before it builds to the boiling point. Often, something as simple as a brisk walk or other exercise can cool you down nicely. Other ways to cope with negative feelings are meditation and yoga. Friends, family, and community associates can help you build a personal buoyancy and foster a sense of well-being.

There is evidence that religious beliefs, such as attending services, praying, and reading religious texts, help to maintain lower stress levels while also contributing to a healthier immune system, and may even endow a longer life. The sense of social connectedness in the community that religion provides can also help to minimize stress and support positive mental health.

Humor can be a beneficial way to insulate yourself from stress. A good laugh triggers the release of endorphins (described on page 294), and can even reduce pain and act as a muscle relaxer. It also can help the body become more resistant to infection while boosting energy levels. Find humor in your daily life. Rent an old *Charlie Chaplin* or *Marx Brothers* video (or other entertainers fitting your tastes) and enjoy it. Learn to laugh at your own mistakes! Such experiences can contribute to a positive and open attitude toward life.

A common form of stress for an older couple is discord between partners. Work on problems with your partner and talk about your feelings when you're both calm. Studies show that positive social interaction, including sexual activity for those who desire it, lowers the level of stress hormones in the blood, helps preserve mental functions, and prevents depression. Review the suggestions dealing with conflict at the end of Chapter 18, *Personality Differences and Styles of Conflict.*

Having a pet dog or cat that you can stroke, talk to, and play with can reduce stress and lower your pulse rate. Walking your dog regularly gives needed exercise. You can chat with other dog owners, or just with those who stop to admire your pet, thus developing new social ties.

Find a way to reduce stress that suits you, and put it to work in your day-to-day life. If stress, tension, or anxiety feels overwhelming, consider consulting a qualified counselor.

SUFFICIENT SLEEP

The human body functions within a natural, daily biological rhythm of activity and rest, just as our environment alternates between sunlight and darkness. Our rest portion, in the form of sleep, not only renews the body but also strengthens the immune system, thus reducing susceptibility to possible infection. Habitual sleep for 6–8 hours within a routine schedule is important. Often a brief afternoon nap can serve to refresh and renew the body and mind for further daytime activities, although too long a nap could detract from uninterrupted nighttime sleep.

If you have trouble getting to sleep or having a satisfactory night's sleep, consider these suggestions before using over-the-counter or prescription medications:

- Go to bed and get up on a regular schedule.
- Avoid eating a heavy meal close to bedtime.
- Do not have an alcoholic drink within two hours of bedtime.
- Do not drink much liquid, including caffeinated beverages, before retiring.
- Relax shortly before bedtime with quiet activities—reading, listening to music, watching "calming" television, or even taking a warm bath, so that your mind is not too stimulated.
- Exercise in the late afternoon or early evening can increase deep sleep that night. A light walk an hour before bedtime can be beneficial.
- If you are unable to fall asleep after 20 minutes, get up, move around, and until you feel sleepy, do a relaxing activity or a quiet, necessary chore.

For further information about achieving good quality sleep, see the two sources at the end of *Internet Health Sources* on page 320.

KEEPING AN ACTIVE MIND

As one ages, short-term memory declines and reaction time lengthens, while the ability to receive and process information slows. Like the effects of physical exercise on the body, mental exercise can help to preserve intellectual ability. Adults who stay mentally active continue to build brain cells and their connections, thus protecting them from the loss of their mental processing ability. Do this with a variety of intellectually stimulating activities. This *cannot* be done if a person sits passively watching television programs for hours each day. Reading interesting literature, solving crossword puzzles, and playing card games or Scrabble, all require mental exercise. Other activities include learning a new language or a musical instrument, attending stimulating classes, assisting in community projects that require active participation and decision-making, maintaining social contacts with family members and close friends, researching and writing a family history, and above all, interacting with an intelligent partner, can encourage mental alertness. Consider learning to use a computer if you have not yet done so. Broaden your knowledge by finding sites on the Internet to obtain information about subjects of interest while communicating with others having similar pursuits. These are all ways of challenging your mind.

You no doubt have many other ideas for engaging in stimulating mental activities. *Four* key factors can give you ongoing support for effective intellectual functioning: (1) finding interesting, challenging activities in which to engage; (2) receiving cooperation and support for your endeavors from other persons; (3) being physically fit, thus contributing to your mental agility; and (4) having a belief in your own intellectual ability to do things that can lead to successful accomplishments and personal satisfaction.

AVOIDING AND OVERCOMING DEPRESSION

The International Longevity Center reports that 20% of people 65 or older suffer from symptoms of depression (*Time* magazine, January 29, 2001, page G4). These symptoms include feelings of fatigue, emptiness, or despair; irritability; lack of concentration; loss of appetite; or sleeplessness. If any of these symptoms are severe or long lasting, or if they interfere with day-to-day functioning, consult your physician or a licensed psychotherapist.

There is evidence that depression can be overcome with many of the activities for a healthy lifestyle that already have been described in this chapter, especially physical exercise, not smoking, getting sufficient sleep, and keeping an active mind. Establishing and pursuing personal goals, while structuring one's everyday life, are vital to maintaining good mental health.

PREVENTIVE MEDICATION

While the practices described here can help most older adults lead a healthy, productive, and enjoyable life, some situations obviously require medical attention. Certain drugs can now be used to prevent or control common medical problems. In postmenopausal women, hormone replacement therapy (HRT), usually a combination of estrogen and some form of progestin can reduce the risk of osteoporosis (reduction in bone density with increased brittleness) and heart disease. Doctor-supervised use of melatonin may be helpful for certain types of insomnia, and testosterone may restore sex drive in people with abnormally low testosterone levels (which may occur in both men and women).

When lifestyle changes fail to lower blood pressure and total cholesterol, drug therapy should be considered. Diuretics are usually the first choice for high blood pressure, whereas statins are generally chosen for high cholesterol. You can take half a regular aspirin tablet (160 mg) every other day, or a baby aspirin (80 mg) every day to reduce the risk of heart disease, and possibly colon and rectal cancers. Many forms of depression are caused not only by life's changes, such as the loss of a loved one, but can be organic in origin due to a chemical imbalance in the brain. Certain medications, such as Prozac™ and Zoloft™ can be very helpful. Check with your doctor for an analysis and recommendation of any medications.

JUDGE YOURSELF

The guidelines and suggestions offered in this chapter can contribute to aging well. They cannot, however, cover all topics or fit all specific needs that you may have. Evaluate your own situation by answering the questions in the following exercise. Think over your responses, deciding what changes you need to make. Then acquire more information or clarifications from readings (see the references starting on page 316), talking with knowledgeable persons, and observing how others handle these lifestyle behaviors. You'll be rewarded with practices that can contribute to a longer, more satisfying life.

SELF-EVALUATION EXERCISE

Carefully answer the following questions. Add notes for yourself and reminders for how to improve your behaviors, possibly from suggestions in this chapter.

1. When you enter a building and need to go to the second floor, do you walk up rather than take the elevator?

   ___ Yes ___ No

2. Are you presently engaged in a beneficial amount of physical exercises?

   ___ Yes ___ No

3. If you are exercising, which type(s) are you doing?

   ____ Endurance ____ Strength ____ Stretching

4. With what exercise(s) would you like to extend your present activities?

5. Examine the following *USDA Daily Food Guide Pyramid* designed for an average 1,600 calories a day, weighted toward a vegetarian diet. (For further details, check the components for a healthy diet on page 297.) Analyze your present diet in terms of the food groups on each level.

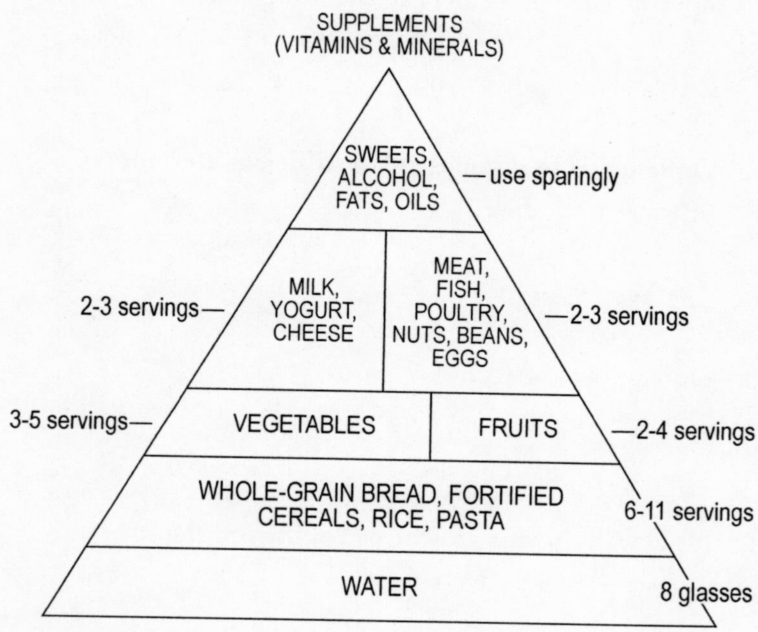

How do you judge yourself? What would you change?

6. Do you usually read (and understand) the nutritional information on food product labels?

___ Yes ___ No

7. If you take dietary supplements, how have you decided what vitamins and minerals to include and in what amounts?

8. What is your daily alcohol consumption?

   Is this acceptable to you? ___ Yes ___ No

9. Do you feel that you drink a sufficient amount of water each day?

   ___ Yes ___ No

10. Do you use tobacco?

    ___ Yes ___ No

11. How well do you protect yourself from the sun?

12. How do you rate yourself in avoiding or controlling stress?

13. How many hours a day do you sit and watch television?

    Is this acceptable? ___ Yes ___ No

14. Do you get sufficient undisturbed sleep at night? If not, what might you do?

15. In what ways do you mentally stimulate yourself?

16. What other intellectual activities might you like to engaged in?

17. Do you have symptoms of depression?

    ___ Yes ___ No

    If so, what might you do to overcome them?

18. Have you found the need for preventive medication? If so, are you careful to follow the routine for proper use?

19. What is your overall judgement of your present lifestyle in terms of the categories and information in this chapter?

    What specific changes might you consider making?

REFERENCES

The Cleveland Clinic Heart Advisor,
P.O. Box 420235,
Palm Coast, FL 32142-0235.

Consumer Reports on Health, P.O. Box 56356,
Boulder, CO 80322-6356;
Telephone: 800-234-2188.

Environmental Nutrition: The Newsletter of Food, Nutrition, and Health, P.O. Box 420451,
Palm Coast, FL 32142-0451.

Fitness After 50*: *It's Never Too Late to Start!
(1996), by Walter Ettinger, Jr., and others;
Pasadena, CA: Beverly Cracom.

Focus on Healthy Aging, P.O. Box 420235,
Palm Coast, FL 32142-0235.

Harvard Men's Health Watch, P.O. Box 420099,
Palm Coast, FL 32142-0099.

Harvard Women's Health Watch, P.O. Box 420068,
Palm Court, FL 32142-0068.

John Hopkins Medical Letter: Health After 50,
Subscription Dept., P.O. Box 420179,
Palm Coast, FL 32142-0179.

***Live Now Age Later*: *Proven Ways to Slow Down the Clock*,** (2000), by Isadore Rosenfeld; New York: Warner Books.

***Living to 100: Lessons in Living to Your Maximum Potential at Any Age*,** (1999), by Thomas Perls and Margery Silver; New York, Basic Books.

***National Institute on Aging (NIH)*,** P.O. Box 8057, Gaithersburg, MD 20898-8057; Telephone: 800-222-2225.

Exercise: A Guide From the National Institute on Aging (1999), NIH Pub. No 99-4258 (also available is a companion exercise video).

In Search of the Secrets of Aging (1996), NIH Pub. No 93-2756.

***Nutrition Action Health Letter*,** Center for Science in the Public Interest, Suite 300, 1875 Connecticut Ave. NW, Washington, DC 20009-5728.

Stealing Time: New Science of Aging (1999), a 3-hour video recording, Public Broadcasting System, 1320 Braddock Place, Alexandria, VA 22314.

Super Nutrition After 50 (1999), by Denise Webb and Elizabeth Ward; Lincolnwood, IL: Publications International Ltd.

University of California, Berkeley Wellness Letter, P.O. Box 420148, Palm Coast, FL 32142.

INTERNET HEALTH SOURCES

www.agingwell.state.ny.us

Described as "a health and wellness village for mature adults with information on eating well, fitness, pharmacy services, health, and safety."

www. andrus.org

AARP website that provides cutting-edge information about living healthy and well.

www.DrWeil.com

This well-known physician provides medical information about herbs and other alternative medicine techniques.

www.fitnesslink.com

News about fitness and starting an exercise program.

www.healthatoz.com

Search engine for health information with more than 50,000 professionally reviewed links and 50 message boards for health-related discussions.

www.healthfinder.gov

Gateway to government and other health-news sites, including the evaluation of information and reporting online health scams.

www.intelihealth.com

General health news and participation by e-mail regarding topics such as cancer, nutrition, and allergies.

www.mayohealth.org

Provides information from the Mayo Clinic about numerous medical subjects, drugs, and a glossary of health jargon.

www.onhealth.com

Local health data such as pollen counts and ultraviolet ray indices. Users can receive e-mail with health news about a particular topic.

www.quackwatch.com

Information about bogus health treatments and ways to spot such a website.

www.yourhealth.com

Information about healthy recipes and being able to question experts regarding health topics.

www.nhlbi.nih.gov/about/ncsdr

Information from the National Center on Sleep Disorders Research; Telephone 301-435-0199.

www.sleepfoundation.org

Information from the National Sleep Foundation that contains research reports and lists of sleep treatment centers.

Chapter 26

FINANCIAL AND LEGAL DOCUMENTS, PROCEDURES, AND RELATED MATTERS

This chapter is a brief orientation to documents and procedures that may be useful as an older couple considers their own financial and legal situation. A list of references is included at the end of the chapter. You can acquire further information and make important decisions in consultation with financial and legal advisors. But first, try your hand at answering these questions.

1. What are the financial advantages and disadvantages of marrying?
2. Why should you have a will?
3. What is the difference between a will and a living trust?
4. What is a durable power of attorney, and how does it differ from a power of attorney for health care?
5. What are the reasons for acquiring title to property as tenants in common or as joint tenants?
6. Do you recognize the benefits for having a nuptial agreement?

7. What are the alternatives available for retirement living facilities?

8. Should you consider acquiring long-term-care insurance?

Were you able to answer each question with confidence and hopefully with correct information? Understanding the topics might be important to you now or in the future. As you proceed through the chapter, see how your answers match the information presented.

FINANCIAL CONSIDERATIONS INFLUENCING WHY OLDER COUPLES MAY OR MAY NOT MARRY

There are a number of financial advantages for couples to live together without marriage. A major reason is that when each person has a sizable income, the couple, filing jointly, may find themselves shifted to a higher tax bracket. This is known as the *marriage penalty.* (Since the time of this writing, action by the Congress may change this regulation). A new marriage also can mean the forfeiture of a deceased spouse's pension rights and medical coverage.

Two single persons living together may find that their separate Social Security benefits are subject to less taxation than they would have if they were married. If a spouse dies and you remarry before age 60, you may lose any benefits due, whereas, usually there is no loss if you wait until your sixtieth birthday to remarry. (This is why **Gayle** is holding off her marriage to **Jim** until she would be 60 years old.)

Another reason for remaining single is that a married couple would need to expend a significant portion of their jointly owned assets before Medicaid would pay the long-term nursing-home-care cost for a sick spouse. The assets of the healthy partner of an unmarried couple are not counted in the eligibility criteria for the ill person.

Often partners do not marry for the above reasons. The Census Bureau indicates that the percentage of cohabiting, unmarried couples has doubled since 1980, and older couples are comprising a large share of this number. It is estimated that in the United States in early 1995, 370,000 men and women over 65 lived together without marriage (*Money* magazine, July 1995), and that number probably has grown since then.

On the other hand, we should not neglect some of the material advantages for being married:

- If you have lived in your home for at least two years, you can sell it and keep up to $250,000 in profit, tax free. For a married couple, the exclusion is $500,000.

- Social Security, company benefits and pension plans, inheritances, and other monetary advantages exist for married couples. (Be sure to add your spouse to your retirement plan as soon as you marry, or you may face a financial penalty.)

- If one married member has significantly more income to draw from than the other, the spousal deduction grants income tax benefits.

- Estate inheritance taxes are avoided because of the unlimited marital deduction on the death of a spouse.

- If one person has health insurance as part of retirement benefits, the spouse can be added. (This also should be done very soon after marriage, or there could be a delay penalty.)

While considering financial advantages and disadvantages of being married, such material concerns should be weighed against other issues. Do you have moral and religious convictions about marriage versus living together? Or, do your feelings about commitment and the meaning of marriage outweigh financial considerations? How serious is the financial loss, if there is one? You and your partner need to discuss these issues.

WILLS

A will is a legal document that must be followed in disposing of a person's properties and debts following death. If you die without a will, the laws of your state decide how these matters will be handled. Everything you own could go to your new spouse. Then, when your spouse dies, everything would go to his or her family, not to your children. Because state community-property laws guide inheritance only for married couples, it is particularly important for unmarried couples to have wills or a trust. An executor, named in the will, handles distribution of the estate's assets to the heirs.

In order for a will to be valid, it must be executed in compliance with the law, including signatures of witnesses. Review your will periodically and especially whenever a new, significant life event occurs. If you wish to revoke or change a will, it can be superseded by a new will, or you can make changes through a hand written and witnessed codicil.

A will that is established if you already have a revocable living trust (see trust section) is called a Pourover Will. If you do not have a trust, it is simply called a will. A pourover will states that your assets are to be distributed by the trust. The advantages of a pourover will is that if you neglected to put something in the trust, it can be distributed as the will provides. Items that have no title, such as jewelry, furniture, artwork, or clothing, can be listed in your pourover will. (Stocks, bonds, real property, and even an automobile with a pink ownership slip have titles and can be included in a trust.)

POWER OF ATTORNEY FOR HEALTH CARE (Sometimes Called a Living Will)

This document provides instructions for medical care if you become terminally ill and unable to express your wishes. It answers such questions as "Do you want pain medication or invasive procedures?" "Do you want to be kept alive through life support?" A living will allows you to appoint someone to be your decision-maker if you cannot speak for yourself. This document can help relieve emotional stress for relatives who may be required to make painful decisions. It is particularly important for committed couples who are *not* married. I knew when I was living with Jerry before we married that should he become ill, I would have had absolutely no say as to his care without such a document.

Be sure that the original, signed form is either given to the person named to act for you, or that the individual knows where it is kept. Also provide a copy for your doctor.

DURABLE POWER OF ATTORNEY FOR FINANCIAL MATTERS

This document authorizes someone you specify to act for you if you should become mentally incapacitated and unable to take actions yourself. It gives the authorized person (called an attorney-in-fact) the right to handle your estate and make financial decisions on your behalf. The term *durable* is included because the authorization remains valid even if the signer (you) becomes legally incompetent to act. Your attorney-in-fact has the right to handle financial matters for you in an emergency, including if you are out of the country. Only assets not in your trust can be handled through this authorization for durable power of attorney.

TRUSTS

Living Trust

A trust is similar to a will, with certain important differences. While a will takes effect when a person dies, a living trust can be set up and used to manage assets during one's lifetime. It is common for the trustor (the person setting up the trust) and the trustee (the person managing the trust) to be the same person. Almost any assets can be placed in a trust – bank accounts, investments, real estate, life insurance, and personal property. When establishing a trust, you change the name or title of each asset to the name of the trust, often with you and your spouse as initial trustees, along with a specified successor trustee. (Example: *Kemp Living Trust, Jerrold E. Kemp, Trustee, Edith Ankersmit Kemp, Trustee, and Andrew Baker, Successor Trustee.*) Then you as trustee, can manage the assets in your trust during your lifetime.

With a trust, the person gives the designated successor trustee power to continue handling the assets even long after death. A will is a public record for anyone to see and requires that the estate pass through the court probate process before the assets can be assigned to the designated heirs. A trust provides *total privacy* and *avoids probate*—the trust's most important, beneficial features. Going through the legal process of probate is costly and can take many months.

A trust is of value for persons on all economic levels. Various types of trusts are available to serve different purposes. A trust may be *revocable,* meaning its terms may be amended, or it is *irrevocable,* in which case it cannot be changed or altered in any way. Consult with a professional advisor to determine if your estate plan can be enhanced by the creation of a trust. It takes time to create a trust and may require a sizable legal fee, although it often is less than the cost to your heirs of going through probate after your death.

Testamentary Trust

This type of trust is created in a will and takes effect upon the death of the person who funds it with estate assets. Like a revocable living trust, your assets can be distributed as you choose. This is less expensive to set up, being part of your will, but it can be much more expensive and time consuming for your heirs after your death because it does not avoid probate.

Charitable Remainder Trust

This trust can be either in your will or in your living trust. It allows a person, while still alive, to leave a specified part of an estate to a favorite charity or nonprofit agency. The recipient pays the individual any income received from the investment, with reduced or eliminated state taxes, for the rest of his or her life. Then, on the person's death, the agency takes ownership of the investment. Another type of charitable remainder trust takes effect after the death of your heirs and saves only estate taxes.

Trusts and the durable power of attorney document should be reviewed and updated as necessary, along with your will, every five years or so. The documents, if not given to the person designated to handle your financial affairs, should be filed with your personal papers.

TENANCIES

If you and your partner, either married or unmarried, are considering buying a home together, you should decide how to hold this property.

Joint Tenants with Right of Survivorship

Shares held in an account are undivided and owned equally by the individuals whose names appear on the property (often spouses and/or children). Upon the death of one owner, ownership passes to the remaining asset owner(s). So if a husband and wife are joint tenants of a house, upon the death of one spouse, the property goes to the other. This transfer of assets avoids probate, but estate taxes will be due. A trust or will does not affect or control this equal distribution.

Tenants in Common

Here assets may be held by two or more people, who are the tenants in common (not necessarily owning equal shares). When one owner dies, as stipulated in the person's will, the deceased person's portion of the assets pass only to his or her heirs, such as children or grandchildren, rather than to the other tenant(s) in common (usually the spouse). Assets within the estate that are held by tenants in common *do not avoid* probate.

Tenancy by the Entirety

This agreement specifies that when property is owned together by a married couple, one spouse cannot terminate the other's rights except by divorce or consent. The assets of one spouse are protected from the creditors of the other spouse. This tenancy is only in effect in some states.

COMMUNITY PROPERTY

In eight states, property acquired during the marriage is considered jointly owned. If one spouse dies, the property automatically goes to the survivor, even if only one spouse is listed as the owner.

PROVISION FOR A PARTNER

You may provide in your will or trust that your partner can remain in a home you own until his or her death, after which the property passes to your heirs. You may also specify that this is in effect only if your partner actually continues to live in the home and does not remarry. (**Barbara**, who leaves her home to her daughter, gives **Leonard** the right to live in it until his death.)

NUPTIAL AGREEMENTS

An agreement between two persons prior to their marriage is most often called a premarital or prenuptial agreement. It specifies what will happen to assets in the event of a death. The agreement is used to accomplish one or more purposes:

- Specify property and assets that each person brings to the marriage that will continue to remain his or her separate property.

- Avoid the effect of the community-property law in states having such laws. The chief advantage here is if a partner is still working, earnings remain under his or her control rather than becoming community property.

A premarital agreement must be in writing and signed by both parties. It should be recorded in the county in which the property affected by the agreement is located.

During a marriage, it is common for assets to become community property, jointly owned by both spouses. But a postnuptial agreement also can be made between a husband and wife. It serves the same purposes as does a prenuptial agreement in keeping assets separate.

RETIREMENT LIVING FACILITIES

While many older couples continue to live in their own houses, condominiums, or rental apartments, the time may come when such independent living is no longer feasible. Some alternative must be found. Following are the kinds of senior retirement homes and communities commonly available.

Retirement Communities

Residences are purchased from a developer, an association, or a prior owner, and monthly dues pay for normal upkeep, repairs, and services. These communities range from private homes, senior apartments, and condominiums in gated communities to mobile-home parks. While such a residence may be considered costly, the facility provides privacy along with extensive recreational and social activities. Usually a planned adult community does not directly offer medical care or meal services, although some offer private, on-call medical service or convenient transportation to such facilities. An inviting restaurant often is on the grounds. **Naomi** and **David**, **Edna** and **Seymour**, and **Nancy** and **Pat** live in such a community.

Congregate Living Facility

A step toward additional care can be to rent rather than purchase a residence. This is usually an apartment where housekeeping services, group meals, and planned activities for residents are provided. Many facilities include transportation to nearby city shopping and medical services. Health qualifications for residents include being ambulatory (mobile and not confined to bed), while some provide a degree of "one-to-one" attention. Private, on-call medical care may be offered. **Mary** and **Fred**, and **Laura** and **Ed** live in such a residence.

Residential Facility

The next step toward more care is designed for individuals who are advanced in age or quite frail, but are still ambulatory. Such a facility usually is licensed and supervised by a state agency. It provides all the services of a congregate living facility as well as daily help such as monitoring medication, aid with bathing, and help with personal tasks. No onsite medical care is offered, but private care is on call. Monthly fees are appreciably higher than those for a congregate facility.

Long-Term-Care Facilities

As with retirement living facilities, there can be different types of long-term-care facilities. The least costly is custodial care, which provides assisted services for persons with limited or no ambulatory ability for such things as getting out of bed, eating, bathing, and walking, but does not require qualified health professionals. A second level builds on custodial care and is intermediate care that may require a qualified nurse, but for limited purposes.

The most comprehensive and expensive program is skilled nursing care for life. It is usually prescribed by a medical doctor and provides services of qualified nurses on a 24-hour basis. There is an initial entrance cost and a monthly rental charge. Often a contract is required, and applicants must demonstrate the ability to meet all financial requirements. Subsidized rates for individuals with limited or fixed retirement income, or qualification for Medicaid after assets are exhausted, may be acceptable. Also, most long-term-care facilities require an initial health examination, and admission is dependent on the results.

Convalescent clinic or hospital service would be available to residents on a temporary basis during illness. If a resident becomes so ill as to be unable to function in the facility, he or she would be moved to a hospital or hospice care.

LONG-TERM-CARE INSURANCE

The average nursing-home care can reach $60,000 a year. Therefore, extended, expensive nursing-home care or home health care can quickly wipe out an individual's or a family's financial assets. While governmental support for long-term-care is being considered by lawmakers, at present, each individual or family must make their own decision regarding purchase of long-term-care insurance.

While such insurance can protect against the high cost of health care, it is not needed by everyone. If you can afford to pay for your own care, it may not be worth the premium expense. An exception might be if you want to protect your assets to pass them to heirs or to charities. Individuals with few assets and low income probably would quickly qualify for governmental assistance through Medicaid. Persons with modest assets and average income are the ones most in need of long-term-care insurance. Many retirement plans and major insurance companies make this protection available.

If you decide that this insurance protection is important, generally you should consider buying it when you are between the ages of 55 and 63. For example, a premium might be about $2,100 a year at age 63 while it is $5,500 at age 75 (costs are at the time of writing this chapter). Carefully consider the terms of a policy, including its length (for your lifetime or for a set number of years), options for home care or nursing-home care, and other conditions or restrictions. Inflation protection can be beneficial if cost rise in the future is anticipated.

To protect their inheritance and peace of mind, some children are purchasing long-term-care policies for their parents. Children in their prime-earning years may be more likely to have adequate cash flow to meet these costs than their asset-rich parents have when now living on limited fixed incomes.

Finally, a report in the *AARP Bulletin* (July–August 1999, page 7) and supported by articles in *Money* magazine and *U.S. News and World Report* magazine indicate that most Americans over age 65 live independently, with fewer than 5 percent in nursing homes, while those reaching the age of 85 eventually need long-term care. But consider the following facts; they could influence your decision about purchasing long-term-care insurance.

- Average nursing-home stay is 2½ years.
- 90% of patients stay less than four years in a long-term-care facility.
- Only Alzheimer's patients tend to have longer-than-average stays.

For professional help with the legal, financial, and related matters treated in this chapter, contact an accountant, financial planner, or lawyer who is familiar with senior-citizen matters. In some communities, the services of a geriatric-care manager may be available. Also, check the references that follow.

REFERENCES

AARP Publications (AARP Fulfillment, 601 E Street NW, Washington, DC 20049).

A Consumers Guide to Probate (stock number 13822).

Getting Married After 50 (Investment Programs Financial Library).

Organizing Your Future: A Guide To Decision-Making in Your Later Years (stock number D13877).

Product Report: Wills and Living Trusts (stock number D14535).

Tomorrow's Choices: Preparing Now for Future Legal, Financial, and Health Care Decisions (stock number D13479).

American Bar Association Legal Guide for Older Americans, American Bar Association Commission on Legal Problems for the Elderly, 7449 15th St. NW, Washington, DC 20005-1022.

All New Avoiding The Medicaid Trap: How To Beat the Catastrophic Costs of Nursing Home Care (1995), by Armond Budish; New York: Henry Holt and Co.

The Elder Law: A Legal and Financial Guide to Later Life (1996), by Peter J. Strauss and Nancy M. Lederman; New York: Facts on File, Inc.

Financial Fitness for Living Together (1996), by Elizabeth Lewin; New York: Facts on File, Inc.

Financial Self-Defense for Unmarried Couples: How to Gain Financial Protection Denied by the Law (1994), by Larry Elkin; New York: Doubleday.

For Better or Worse? A Legal and Financial Guide to Marriage (1992), by Johnette Duff and George G. Truitt; Orlando, FL: Legalines.

How To Avoid Probate! (1993), by Norman F. Dacey; New York: HarperCollins.

Leaving Money Wisely: Creative Estate Planning for Middle- and Upper-Income Americans (1993), by David W. Belin; Old Tappin, NJ: Simon & Schuster.

The Living Together Kit: A Legal Guide for Unmarried Couples (1994), by Toni Ihara and Ralph Warner; Berkeley, CA: Nolo Press.

Living Trusts and Simple Ways to Avoid Probate (1998), by Karen Ann Rolcik; Naperville, IL: Sourcebooks.

Love After 50: The Complete Legal and Financial Guide (1994), by Johnette Duff and George Truitt; Orlando, FL: Love and Money Press.

Make Your Own Living Trust (1990), by Denis Clifford; Berkeley, CA: Nolo Press.

Plan Your Estate: Absolutely Everything You Need to Know to Protect Your Loved Ones (1998), by Denise Clifford and Cora Jordan. Berkeley; CA: Nolo Press,

Planning for Incapacity: A Self-Help Guide to Advance Directives, Legal Counsel for the Elderly, Inc. P.O. Box 96474, Washington, DC 20090.

Understanding Living Trusts: How To Avoid Probate, Save Taxes, and More (1990), by Vickie Schumacher and Jim Schumacher; Santa Monica, CA: Schumacher & Co.

Useful Websites

www. aarp.org
www.elderweb.com
www.longtermcareinsurance.org
www.ushc-online.org
(United Seniors Health Cooperative)
www.nolo.com (Internet site at the Self-Help Law Center from Nolo Press; includes legal tips to help non-traditional families plan for the future)

CONCLUDING THOUGHTS

It has been a deeply enriching experience to interview the couples whose stories fill this book. Their joys and struggles confirm my own experiences with my husband Jerry, mirroring the opening lines of my wedding vows:

I never thought that love would come to me
so strongly, so late in life.

I am indeed blessed.

Our bodies may age, our memories may slip a little, but our hearts remain the same. The capacity to love deeply and to be as sexually active as health allows do not change. In fact, with added maturity and the awareness that time is limited, each present moment is precious.

THE CAPACITY TO GROW AND CHANGE

The ability to learn and grow continues throughout life. Some of the couples interviewed had stable, happy childhoods and good, long first marriages. After a period of being widowed, they now experience successful later life relationships. But others had difficult, sometimes horrendous childhoods and painful earlier marriages. Yet, in learning from these experiences, they also were able to form satisfying later unions.

One benefit of a new, older relationship is that it gives individuals the chance to find personal strengths not previously developed. A loving partnership provides a safe environment for the freedom to thrive. **Nancy**, in her partnership with **Pat**, found a more confident and sexual self not previously experienced. **Jim**, in his relationship with **Gayle**, enhanced his emotional side. With Jerry, I have learned to be more outgoing and to laugh and play. Jerry has become more openly affectionate and can more easily say, "I love you." We have both become more accepting of each other's ways.

RESPECTING EACH OTHER'S BEINGS

Throughout our stories of older couples, there runs a common thread. In virtually every case of a solid partnership, there is a foundation of mutual acceptance and respect for the other person as he or she is. This means accepting the little quirks and rough edges another individual brings to a relationship. These are the foibles and irritations of life with someone else. Paradoxically, such acceptance provides the safety that makes possible natural, gradual change.

No one likes feeling coerced or criticized. Remember the parent or teacher who demanded changes from you? This triggered resentment, resistance, and anger. But a compassionate request can prompt a change that is freely given as a gift of caring. This process is particularly essential in older couples, when the habits, attitudes, and simple ways of doing things are well established in each person.

A long-term study by psychologists Robert Levenson and John Gottman confirms the importance of this acceptance. In research that spanned more than 20 years, they studied more than a thousand couples, trying to find what keeps them together and what drives them apart. They interviewed 50 couples who had been together for 50 years or more, many of whom were still happily married. When asked by a newspaper reporter what these couples were good at, Dr. Levenson replied, "They are terrific at listening to each other. They have respect for each other's way of being. They are not trying to change each other. And you see it both in the big things like accepting each other's personalities, their strengths and weaknesses, and in the little everyday details of living" (from *The East Bay Express* newspaper, July 9, 1999, page 9).

COMPARING EARLY AND LATE LIFE UNIONS

In his 1986 book, *Vital Involvement in Old Age,* renowned psychologist Eric Erickson speaks of a second chance for love and marriage in the later years. His belief is based on the experiences of a number of his subjects who, although remarried, believed that in heaven they would be reunited with their first spouse. To quote Erickson:

> In the minds of our remarried subjects, marriage in youth and marriage in later life seem to represent two different kinds of intimacy. Marriage in youth appears to imply the fusion of individual identities in mutual intimacy and these people view this fusion as permanent, regardless of the interventions of death or remarriage. In contrast, marriage in later life seems to represent a commitment to companionship. Although that commitment involves intimacy, sacrifice, compromise, and reciprocity, although it may be expected to last for the rest of life, it nonetheless remains separate from the early, intimate fusion that seems to transcend death and time. (Eric Erickson, *Vital Involvement in Old Age,* 1986; New York: W.W. Norton, page 123)

I believe that most young adults in their twenties go into marriage with incomplete identity formations, and therefore, their two identities are more likely to fuse. However, the high divorce rate, especially in young marriages, leads one to question the permanence of the mutual intimacy that Erickson describes.

My late husband and I, married early in life, are an example of the fusion of two identities that worked out well. Gradually over the years, even though we came from two widely different cultures, we grew more and more alike in values, manner of speech, and even in the way we looked and dressed. In contrast, the older individuals I interviewed had developed their own individualities and were able to make compromises in their new relationships without losing their sense of self. They are, as David Schnarel says in his book, *Passionate Marriage*, "differentiated." According to Schnarel, "Differentiation is your ability to maintain your sense of self when you are emotionally and/or physically close to others, especially as they become increasingly important to you" (David Schnarel, *Passionate Marriage*, 1997; New York: An Owl Book, Henry Holt, page 56).

The fact that one can have an intimate relationship at the stage of life where one is "differentiated" is in itself, remarkable and is perhaps, the reason why these older relationships are so joyous.

It is almost impossible to place one life stage of marriage as superior to another. I've often thought that if I should go to heaven, I would have a difficult time choosing between my late husband and Jerry. My earlier marriage was bound not only by the fusion of our two identities, but also by raising a child and many years of living together. Jerry and I have more time and freedom to know and enjoy each other intellectually, emotionally, and sexually. Those interviewed who were widowed after successful long first marriages still did not rate their new relationship as inferior—far from it. I would venture to say that a partnership between two fully developed individuals is at least equal in quality to earlier relationships where identities were fused.

FORMING THE *WE* WHILE PRESERVING THE *I*

Judith Wallerstein, in her book, *The Good Marriage*, speaks of forming a *we*. She sees a young couple as "putting together a shared vision of how they want to spend their lives together—constructing the psychological identity of the marriage as an entity in itself" (Judith Wallerstein, *The Good Marriage*, 1995; New York: Warner Books, page 62).

Individual autonomy and the togetherness of the *we* are not mutually exclusive. A person who is not fully individuated could fear being engulfed by an intimate relationship and see requests for compromise as controlling. The older adult who is differentiated and has a secure sense of self is not threatened by the many compromises needed to form this "we." Still, for the older individual who has been alone for a long time or is not yet emotionally detached from a previous spouse, it may take some time to form the *we*. For example, **Bill** has had difficulty bonding with **Joyce,** as he still idealizes his late wife.

Jerry and I formed this *we* gradually as we lived together. Early in our relationship, I was extremely upset each time Jerry reminded me to turn off a light. I discussed this problem with a good friend, who advised me just to say "thank you" and then turn off the light. I told her that I couldn't gracefully do so, as I would be too angry. Now, a few years later, I find myself saying "thank you" and turning off a light without even realizing it. Jerry, in turn, seems much less concerned with habits of mine that previously annoyed him greatly. These adjustments occurred on an almost unconscious level and have helped us to form a harmonious togetherness without losing our separate individualities.

In every good relationship, there is a balance between the autonomy of the individuals involved and the togetherness that they gradually form. In older couplings, this task can be easier because the partners are already secure in their own sense of self, but it can also be difficult because each person has spent many years forming separate values, attitudes, and habits. **Joanne** and **Andy** vividly illustrate this theme of balancing separateness and togetherness.

THE BONDING OF SEXUALITY

All of our couples were active sexually in the early days of their relationship, no matter what age they first became involved. For most, their first sexual encounter marked the start of their commitment to each other. Many have continued with sexual intercourse very late into life. **Ruth**, age 78, and **Paul**, 80, have sexual activity almost every morning and find the experience "loveable." Those couples whose medical problems interfere with intercourse still express their affection for each other physically, and for almost all those interviewed, some form of sexuality helps to maintain the strong tie between them.

Jerry and I also experience the bonding quality of sex. Our love life leads to much affectionate teasing and laughter, making problems seem less important. Both of us had seriously ill spouses, so our sexual life makes up for long periods of abstinence and adds immeasurably to the *we* between us.

LIVING TOGETHER FIRST ... DOES IT MAKE FOR A MORE SUCCESSFUL OLDER MARRIAGE?

A number of our couples lived together for a period of time before marriage. Others married without previous cohabitation, believing that such an arrangement was contrary to their moral principles or the expectations of family, friends, and neighbors. Considering the age of these couples and the prevailing mores of the times when they were raised, this is understandable. The question is, does cohabiting before marriage make a more successful union?

Judith Wallerstein proposes that many young couples "play" at living together. For a good marriage, she states, "the path depends on the motivations that have brought the couple together, and whether they use the time together to build a relationship that can become a good marriage. If it begins as play, does it remain play or become serious? Does it allow them to learn about themselves and what they do or do not want?" (*The Good Marriage,* page 176)

I believe that the couples interviewed did not "play" at living together. Many years of life and the ups and downs of previous relationships have given them the wisdom to seriously use the time to work out difficulties. Those of our couples who chose to marry after living together see themselves as making a public declaration of their love and commitment. A number of our couples living together have no intention of ever marrying, although they see themselves committed to the relationship for life. This attitude is prevalent among many older couples. Because they do not plan to raise children, they see no reason for marriage. There are also important financial reasons for both marrying and not marrying (see page 322 in Chapter 26). And there are couples, such as **Nancy** and **Pat**, and **John** and **Karin**, who chose to live not only unmarried, but separately, yet in a loving relationship.

If you embarking on a committed relationship, you need to make the important decision of whether you will live together before marriage, or indeed whether to marry at all, based upon your own and your partner's personal values.

THE ABILITY TO LOVE AGAIN

When the first marriage was good and ended in the death of a spouse, those interviewed shed tears when they discussed the relationship with me. But a happy new relationship need in no way negate or diminish the cherished years of an earlier marriage. This is important for both partners in a new relationship to understand, as well as for the grown children of the earlier marriage.

When I spend time in the house where I raised my family, I still have dreams of my late husband. I recently reminisced with my adult daughter about those precious years when we were a young family. She is glad for Jerry and me and is relieved to know that I have not thrown away the past.

Gabriel Marquez, in his novel, *Love in the Time of Cholera,* beautifully describes the ability to love deeply:

> He saw no reason why Fermina Daza should not be a widow, prepared by life to accept him just as he was, without fantasies of guilt because of her dead husband, resolved to discover with him the other happiness of being happy twice, with one love for everyday use which would become, more and more, a miracle of being alive, and the other love that belonged to her alone, the love immunized by death against all contagion. (Gabriel Marquez, *Love in the Time of Cholera,* 1989; New York: Penguin Books, page 203)

If you have the capacity to love, that capacity does not die with your beloved. As many of our couples demonstrate, love can be reignited at any age.

THE ABILITY TO FIND LOVE MISSED IN THE PAST

Many of our couples have found in their new relationship a love never before experienced. They may have had a marriage ending in divorce, or endured an unsatisfactory marriage ending only with the partner's death.

Joanne and **Andy** each had long marriages, ending in divorces, that were lacking in intimacy, affection, and sexuality. These difficult experiences have greatly increased their appreciation of present happiness.

Laura was, for years, in a marriage with a husband who was emotionally distant and sexually unfaithful. She, like many women of her generation, had no financial ability to provide for herself and her children. She was taught not to expect much for herself and to stay in a marriage no matter what. Later in life, after her husband's death, she found in **Ed** a man who offered her fidelity, companionship, and love.

There are so many reasons why an early marriage may be unsatisfactory. Our present older generation received tremendous pressure to marry relatively young. I remember my mother worrying that I would be an "old maid" because I did not find a husband while I was in college. If I had married my college sweetheart, it would have been a disaster. I was too unsure of myself and too immature to make a wise choice. If the partners are immature, there might be a danger of their psyches being so merged that the individuality of one or both could be smothered. This could lead to a spouse leaving the marriage in order to "find" him or herself.

Other early marriages replicate difficult childhood experiences. A little girl may have longed for the love of an emotionally unavailable father. As a young woman, she may choose a husband with similar traits, attempting again in vain to find the love she missed as a child. Harold, described in the chapter, *Are You Ready?* chose a wife much like his mentally unstable mother, and it took him many unhappy years before he gathered the courage to divorce her. Some individuals repeat this pattern over and over again, and have a series of failed relationships. But this is not inevitable. It takes courage, hope, and trust to heal from earlier wounds, but as so many of our couples prove, it is possible to choose wisely in later life and find the love they missed in the past.

DOES AN OLDER WOMAN STAND A CHANCE?

Many women reading this book will say to themselves, "This is all very nice, but there are so many more older women than men that I don't stand a chance of finding a partner." Unfortunately, it is much more difficult for an older woman to become involved in a new relationship. Victoria Jaycox, author of *Single Again: A Guide for Women Starting Over,* states: "An informal estimate given to me by the demographer Martha Farnsworth Riche put the gap between the number of women who would want a marriage and the number of men they might want to marry at as much as ten or even twenty to one." Then she concludes, "after a certain age, finding someone great to marry is like winning the office pool" (Victoria Jaycox, *Single Again: A Guide for Women Starting Over,* 1999; New York: W.W. Norton, page 246).

With the odds against me, in my own life, I feel lucky to have found Jerry. For Jerry, being a man, finding a mate was much easier. Two years after his wife's death, he began actively searching for a new partner. He had no doubt that he would find someone. He was simply selective as to common interests, religion, and physical attractiveness. In the four years that I had been alone before meeting Jerry, I was often lonely and wanted a compatible partner. I was by no means sure that I would find one. I joined a social group for older singles in which the ratio was approximately ten women to every man and I belonged to several hiking clubs, where again, there were many more women than men. I learned, as did most of my single women friends, to be content with enjoyable activities and closeness with family and friends.

Certainly, if an older woman wants a new relationship, she could do all that's suggested in Section Three of this book entitled, *How Do You Find a Partner?* But she needs to also find fulfillment in her single life. And paradoxically, by accepting her single state, and being an active and interesting woman, she is much more likely to find a suitable partner.

YOUNG-OLD AND OLD-OLD

The couples interviewed cover a wide range of ages and length of time they had been together. **Joanne**, age 59, and **Andy**, 60, are one of our youngest couples. They dated 14 months and have been living together for 8 months. On the opposite end of the spectrum are **Laura**, age 80, and **Ed**, 90. With our older couples, we have the advantage of seeing changes over time. Laura and Ed married when they were 61 and 71, respectively, and thus, have been together 19 years. They both are experiencing health problems that limit their activities, with Ed's being particularly severe. Despite these limitations, they continue to find joy in life and in each other's company.

Mary Pipher, in her recent book, *Another Country: Navigating the Emotional Terrain of our Elders,* makes a distinction between *young-old* and *old-old* with these words:

> My own belief is that loss of health is what delineates the two stages of old age. Until people lose their health, they are in the young-old category. Until people are ill, many keep their old routines and add some new pleasurable ones. Even if they lose their spouses they still can enjoy friends and family. Retired people travel, do volunteer work, pursue

> creative activities, and play cards or golf. However, poor health changes everything.
>
> In America, the young-old are mostly in their sixties and seventies. When health falls apart, generally in the mid-seventies or later, the young-old move into the old-old stage. Susan Sontag describes the difference between the two stages of old age this way: "Everyone who is born holds dual citizenship, in the kingdom of the well and in the kingdom of the sick." (Mary Pipher, *Another Country: Navigating the Emotional Terrain of Our Elders,* 1999; New York: Penguin Putnam, page 28)

Couples who start their relationship in the period of *young-old* need to be aware that if they both live long enough, they will eventually, with increasing medical problems, become *old-old*, with all the adjustments that entails. As Bette Davis, the late actress, said, "Old age isn't for sissies." Much loyalty and mutual support are needed in those difficult times.

SOME HELPFUL SUGGESTIONS

What have we learned from the couples who so freely shared their lives, loves, and struggles with me? Here are some thoughts:

- First, it is never too late to be in love.

- There needs to be a certain amount of negotiation and change in an older couple's union, but it is essential to have a deep internal acceptance of your partner as he or she is.

- In every good, older relationship, there is a balance between togetherness and separateness, and this balance varies with each couple.

- Sexual satisfaction is possible throughout life. Age is no barrier.

- Your loving partnership is more important than any small issues that bother you. Conflict is inevitable in all relationships, but avoid blaming, calling names, and threatening to leave. Take a "time out" until you both are able to discuss issues calmly. Don't hold grudges.

- A sense of humor can make problems seem much smaller, and it helps keep a spark alive in an older relationship.

- Accept that your partner has had previous loves. It is good to be able to share freely your past lives with each other without undue jealousy.

- Your children and grandchildren may or may not accept your new partner. Keep in mind that the relationship with your mate needs to be primary.

- Early in your relationship, discuss financial arrangements, particularly how expenses will be shared. In time, consider to whom each will leave his or her assets, the advisability of Power of Attorney for Health Care, long-term-care insurance, and alternatives for various types of retirement living (see Chapter 26).

- When forming a relationship later in life, one of you is likely to eventually become a caretaker. Feelings of resentment are normal. You need not blame yourself as long as your actions are kind and responsible.

- As you and your partner come closer to the end of life, know that you might experience the pain of a loss. Be aware that present joys are worth the pain. Knowing that life is short, live each moment with your loved one to its fullest.

I end this book by again quoting from Gabriel Marques' book, *Love in the Time of Cholera.* Referring to Fermina Daza and her lover, Florentino Ariza, both very along in years, he states:

> For they had lived together long enough to know that love was always love, any time and any place, but it was more solid the closer it came to death. (page 345)

May all the couples interviewed experience such love and joy until the end of their lives together. Whether you are searching for a new coupling or already are involved in an older relationship, may you find a love that grows stronger with each passing year.

Edith Ankersmit Kemp

JERRY'S THOUGHTS

In many chapters Edith has given you her professional analysis and thoughts about our relationship. May I make a few observations?

When we tell friends we are writing a book together, they often question how our marriage has survived this task! Yes, we have had differences and conflicts. But by cooperating, sharing ideas, and even arguing at times, we have become closer. It's a good feeling. As Shakespeare wrote:

I count myself in nothing
else so happy
As in a soul remembering
my good wife.

(King Richard II)

INTERVIEWEE INDEX

The following list indicates pages on which references are made to each of the persons interviewed.

TOPICAL INDEX

The following topics are treated in chapters of Sections Two, Three, and Four. They relate to experiences of the interviewees along with information provided by the authors.